Cardiovascular Disease

The Oxidized Lipid Hypothesis

How to Intervene in the Disease Process

Thomas L. Copmann, M.S., Ph.D.

The author of this book is not a physician and the ideas, procedures, and suggestions in this book are not intended as a substitute for the medical advice of a trained health professional. All matters regarding your health require medical supervision. Consult your physician before adopting the suggestions in this book, as well as about any condition that may require diagnosis or medical attention. The author and publisher disclaim any liability arising directly or indirectly from the use of this book.

Contents

Introduction

Cardiovascular disease (CVD) is a general term used to encompass any disease of the heart and/or blood vessels. These diseases are a group of disorders of the heart and blood vessels including *coronary heart disease* (a disease of the blood vessels supplying the heart), *cerebrovascular disease* (disease of the blood vessels supplying the brain), *peripheral arterial disease* (disease of blood vessels supplying the arms and legs), *rheumatic heart disease* (damage to the heart from rheumatic fever, caused by streptococcal bacteria); *congenital heart disease* (birth defects affecting the development of the heart); and *deep vein thrombosis and pulmonary embolism* (blood clots in the leg veins, which can migrate to the heart and lungs).

In this book we will focus mainly on atherosclerosis which is a disease of the arteries characterized by the deposition of plaques of fatty material on their inner walls. Atherosclerosis is a slow, progressive disease that begins with damage or injury to the inner layer of an artery or endothelium. We will review several hypotheses on the development of CVD, as well as, multiple areas of current research into therapeutic intervention.

Diseases of the heart are currently the leading cause of death across the entire American population, accounting for a third of all deaths and costing the economy over $400 billion per year. In the US, CVD accounts for more deaths than all deaths from cancer combined! One person dies every 37 seconds from CVD, and it is estimated that by 2030, over 1 million people will die from CVD every year in the US.

Globally, cardiovascular diseases are the number one cause of death, with a staggering 17.9 million people dying from CVDs in 2019, representing 32% of all global deaths (World Health Organization).

Age is a major risk factor for cardiovascular disease, along with smoking, diabetes and poor diet. All of these factors have a common feature: they increase the levels of oxidative stress. Much is known regarding oxidative stress, aging and the development of cardiovascular disease, but the precise pathogenesis and mechanisms of this relationship remains complex. While significant progress has been made in the treatment of cardiovascular disease, the incidence continues to increase.

We know that atherosclerosis begins with injury to the endothelial cells lining medium and large arteries. There is significant evidence that suggests exposure to dietary omega-6 polyunsaturated fatty acids can directly affect endothelial cell metabolism. Significant amounts of data have been accumulated to show that polyunsaturated fats can induce discernable injury to endothelial cells in blood vessels. This is the basis of the oxidized lipid hypothesis.

The problem with omega-6 polyunsaturated oils is their molecular structure. Polyunsaturated fats refer to the fact that they have multiple double bonds between carbon atoms. Oxygen reacts with the double bonds in a process called lipid peroxidation. The end result is the formation of highly reactive free radicals which interact with cellular membranes, as well as nuclear DNA, and deplete cells of their antioxidant defenses.

The purpose of this book is not to review treatment protocols, but instead look at the current state of research, hopefully providing the reader a foundation of understanding of cardiovascular disease. As you read the content of this book, I would ask you to keep an open mind, and then make your own decisions based on the totality of information. Some of what you will be presented will be contrary to information you may find on the web. And there is a large gap in understanding at the bedside from what is known in animal studies. This is because clinical trial is lengthy, expensive, and the endpoints (mortality) are difficult to reach in significant numbers.

Hopefully the material within this book will help you understand the progression of CVD, and areas of potential intervention, should you be one of the one in three people with one or more of the cardiovascular diseases.

1. Cardiovascular Disease

Heart disease was for the most part unknown in 1900. In fact, the first journal publication on heart disease did not appear until 1921. Since then, heart disease has increased from 1,000 people in 1910 to 58.5 million in 2005; an increase of 5,820% (Figure 1). Coincidentally, Mazola corn oil and Crisco were introduced in 1911. Prior to 1911, the primary cooking fats were saturated fats from butter and

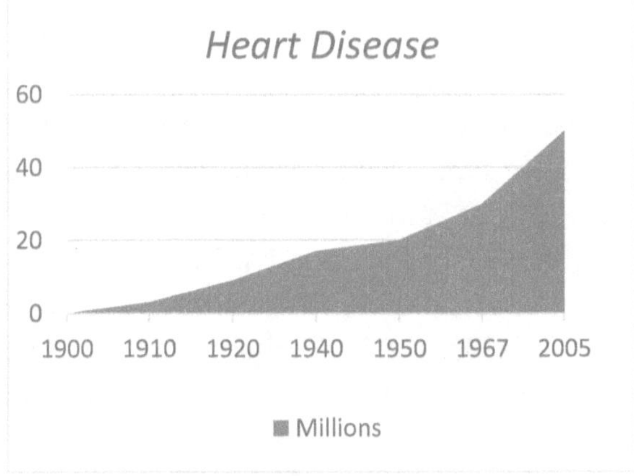

Figure 1: Number of People Diagnoses with Heart Disease 1900 to 2005. Crisco and corn oil were introduced in 1911.

tallow. The intake of omega-6 vegetable oils, particularly soybean oil, began to increase in the USA starting in the early 1900s at a time when the consumption of butter and lard was on the decline. This caused a more than two-fold increase in the intake of linoleic acid, the main omega-6 polyunsaturated fat found in vegetable oils, which now makes up around 8% to 10% of total energy intake in the Western world.

A systematic review of studies measuring the changes in linoleic acid concentration in subcutaneous adipose tissue in the USA revealed an approximate 2.5-fold increase in linoleic acid, increasing from 9.1% to 21.5% from 1959 to 2008. Importantly, the concentration of linoleic acid in adipose tissue is a reliable marker of intake as the half-life of linoleic acid is approximately 2 years in adipose tissue. The authors of the study also noted that the increase in adipose tissue linoleic paralleled the increase in the prevalence of diabetes, obesity and asthma.

As shown in Figure 2, while we are better able to treat heart disease, the prevalence of heart disease continues to rise. By 1950, coronary heart disease, was the leading cause of death in the United States, responsible for more than 30% of all deaths. Myocardial infarction (MI) caused no more than three thousand deaths per year in 1930. By 1960, there were at least 500,000 MI deaths per year in the US.

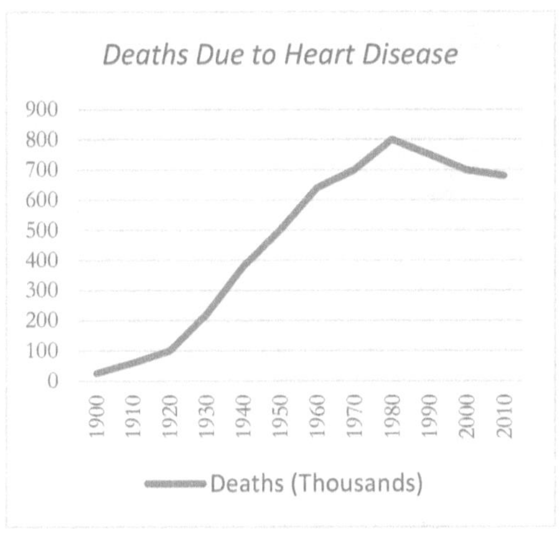

Figure 2: Deaths (In Thousands) Due to Heart Disease.

During that time, research began to solidify around the "cholesterol hypothesis" as the cause of heart disease. To better understand the "cholesterol hypothesis", we need to review the data and assumptions behind it. The hypothesis argues that cholesterol in the blood is deposited in the arteries thereby causing the blockage seen in atherosclerosis. The first published evidence for the cholesterol hypothesis came when German researcher Windaus noted that aortas of patients with atherosclerosis contain more cholesterol in their aortas compared to healthy individuals. The landmark study came in 1913, when Nikolaj Nikolajewitsch Anitschkow fed cholesterol to rabbits causing atherosclerosis. In subsequent work, Anitschkow concluded that the process of atherosclerosis starts with the formation of fatty streaks. However, cholesterol is only soluble in oil so many of these studies used corn oil as the vehicle for administration thereby putting the results in question.

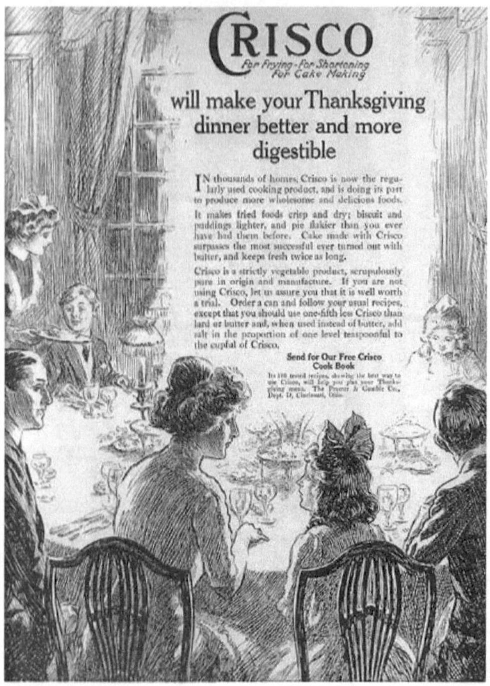

Figure 3: Crisco advertisement November 1912 from the Ladies Home Journal.

Around the same time, the seed oil industry was in crisis. Seed oils were being used in paints and plastics but were being displaced by petroleum-based products. The industry needed new markets, and proposed a marketing strategy that "vegetable" oils were healthier than traditional animal fats. After all, polyunsaturated fats were observed to lower cholesterol blood levels. Crisco, initially made with hydrogenated cottonseed oil, is the quintessential imitation food. (The name Crisco is derived from Crystalized Cottonseed Oil.) Crisco advertisements from the 1900 frequently included health claims. Crisco's first ad campaign introduced the "all-vegetable" shortening as "a healthier alternative to cooking with animal fats." An ad in 1912 claimed "It's digestible" (Figure 3). Crisco was made by hydrogenating cottonseed oil to make a product the resembled lard. Unfortunately, hydrogenation introduces trans fats, the consequences of which were not know at the time.

In 1939, Muller published findings in the *Annals of Internal Medicine* that patients with familial cases of hypercholesterolemia had significantly more cardiovascular disease than people without increased plasma cholesterol levels thereby confirming Anitschkow's earlier work postulating cholesterol is a causal factor in atherosclerosis.

This was the beginning of many studies that supported the cholesterol hypothesis. A 1955 report on artery plaques in soldiers killed during the Korean War received a significant amount of attention. Postmortem examination of remains showed significant development of atherosclerosis despite their young age. They concluded dietary influence had caused early development of atherosclerotic plaques. There were other epidemiological studies showing that Japanese had almost as much pathogenic plaque despite having less animal fats in their diet but these were mostly ignored.

The American Heart Association (AHA) was a relatively obscure association until Procter & Gamble gave $1.5 million from its radio show, *Truth or Consequences*, allowing the organization to go national. The AHA aired a fund raiser in 1956 on all three major networks promoting the "prudent Diet". The panel included renowned researchers at the time and supported the "cholesterol "hypothesis as the cause of the heart disease. However, they went one step further proposing a diet of corn oil, margarine, chicken and cold cereal replacing butter, lard, beef and eggs. Dr. Dudley White, was the lone panelist who disputed his colleagues at the AHA. Dr. White reminded the panel that myocardial infarction was nonexistent in 1900 when corn oil was unavailable and when egg consumption was three times what it was in 1956. Dr. White is quoted as having said: "I began my practice as a cardiologist in 1921 and I never saw an MI patent until 1928. Back in the MI free days before 1920, the fats were butter and lard and I think that we would all benefit from the kind of diet that we had at a time when no one had ever heard the words "corn oil."

This followed with the AHA issuing dietary guidelines in 1957. The 1957 AHA report concluded that there was a causal relationship between saturated fats and the pathogenesis of atherosclerosis.

The food industry quickly took up the banner promoting health benefits of vegetable oils. A Mazola oil ad from 1951 touted "no cholesterol". Another ad made such claims as: "Best for cutting down saturated fats in your diet"; "Polyunsaturates are a plus in Mazola"; "Take this ad to your doctor…" The ad goes on to claim a 17% reduction in serum cholesterol". A major medical journal advertisement recommended Fleishmann's unsalted margarine for patients with high blood pressure.

Ancel Keys, a professor at the University of Minnesota, published his Six Country Analysis in 1953. Keys suggested an association between dietary fat and mortality from heart disease. Critics pointed out that Keys had data for 22 countries, but selected data from just 6. (Keys excluded countries with a high fat diet and low rates of heart disease).

In 1977, the *Select Committee on Nutrition and Human Needs* of the United States Senate published a committee report titled *Dietary Goals for the United States*. The Committee, chaired by George McGovern, sought to "set national dietary goal for the country." The report was released with a press briefing including several prominent nutritional researchers including Dr. Beverly Winikoff (Rockefeller Foundation), Dr. Philip Lee (University of California), Dr. D.M. Hegsted (Harvard), and a handful of Senators. The Committee recommended:

- Increase carbohydrate intake between 55 - 60 percent of calories,
- Decrease dietary fat intake to no more than 30 percent of calories, with a reduction in intake of saturated fat, and recommended approximately equivalent distributions among saturated, polyunsaturated, and monounsaturated fats to meet the 30 percent target,

- Decrease cholesterol intake to 300 mg per day,
- Decrease sugar intake to 15 percent of calories,
- Decrease salt intake to 3 g per day.

The report was met with skepticism from both industry and research community who felt the literature at the time did not support the specific intake goals. Nonetheless, the Department of Agriculture and the Department of Health, Education, and Welfare established a joint committee whose goals were the focus of the controversy that existed among some nutritionists and others concerned with food, nutrition, and health. They collectively published the *Dietary Guidelines for Americans* brochure in February 1980.

At the same time, the FDA *Select Committee on GRAS Substances* (SCOGS) issued their opinion on Hydrogenated soybean oil. The GRAS (Generally Recognized as Safe) ingredient reviews were conducted by the Select Committee in response to a 1969 White House directive by then President Richard M. Nixon. The Select Committee found: "There is no evidence in the available information on hydrogenated soybean oil that demonstrates, or suggests reasonable grounds to suspect, a hazard to the public when it is used as a direct or indirect food ingredient at levels that are now current or that might reasonably be expected in the future." The Committee report was dismissive on the effect of trans-fats. The opinion concluded: "the weight of evidence indicates that trans-monoenoic acids, the principal geometric isomers present in hydrogenated soybean oil, are not hypercholesterolemic. Similarly, the results of animal experimentation indicate that trans-acids of hydrogenated soybean oil are not atherogenic at normal dietary levels." Of course, we now know that is not the case.

The same committee issued their GRAS opinion on coconut oil, peanut oil, and oleic acid in 1975. They found "no evidence in the available information on coconut oil, peanut oil, and oleic acid that demonstrates, or suggests reasonable grounds to suspect, a hazard to the public as they are now used in paper and cotton packaging material for food at levels now current or as they might reasonably be expected to be used for such purposes in the future." Clearly, the FDA did not differentiate between types of oil. They went on to conclude: "There is no evidence in the available information on linoleic acid that demonstrates, or suggests reasonable grounds to suspect, a hazard to the public when it is used as a nutrient or dietary supplement at levels now current or that might reasonably be expected in the future."

In 1968, Paul Leren published *The Effect of Plasma Cholesterol Lowering Diet in Male Survivors of Myocardial Infarction. A Controlled Clinical Trial*. This is the first long term study which supported a reduction in cardiovascular disease with a cholesterol lowering diet. In 1984, the *Lipid Research Clinics Coronary Primary Prevention Trial* results were published supporting the relationship of the incidence of coronary heart disease to cholesterol lowering. This trial showed that cholestyramine, a drug which lowered plasma cholesterol by about 10%, lowered the relative risk of coronary heart disease by almost 20%. Then, in 1994, the well-known *Scandinavian Simvastatin Survival Study Group: Randomized Trial of Cholesterol Lowering in 4444 Patients with Coronary Heart Disease: The Scandinavian Simvastatin Survival Study (4S)* was published in the Lancet. In this study simvastatin (a statin drug) reduced plasma cholesterol levels by approximately 25%, with a reduction in the relative risk of death due to coronary heart disease by 42%.

These studies served to firmly entrench the cholesterol hypothesis. While the American Medical Association initially did not support the hypothesis, the American Heart Association was firmly on board. And in 1961 the AHA advocated the substitution of polyunsaturated oils for saturated fats, despite little evidence to support this statement.

Cracks form in the Cholesterol Hypothesis

Cracks started to develop in the cholesterol hypothesis. In June 1966, Drs. Rose, Thomson, and Williams published an article in the British Medical Journal on the results of a prospective study of corn oil in patients with Ischemic Heart Disease. Patients were equally divided into one of three groups receiving either 80g/day corn oil, or olive oil; or a control group. Patients in both oil groups were instructed to avoid fried foods, fatty meat, sausages, pastry, ice-cream, cheese, cakes, etc. while milk, eggs, and butter were restricted. The oil supplement was divided into three equal doses at meal-times. The patients were followed for two years. The patients receiving corn oil had a significant reduction in total cholesterol, but shockingly had 25% more deaths than either the olive oil or control group! The proportions of patients remaining alive and free of re-infarction (fatal or non-fatal) was greater for the control group (75%) than for the two oil groups (olive oil 57%, corn oil 52%).

And remember the "Prudent Diet" of corn oil, margarine, fish, chicken and cold cereal promoted on national television? The results were published in 1961 in the *Journal of the American Medical Association*. The diet group, had an average serum cholesterol of 220 mg/dl, compared to 250 mg/dl in the meat-and-potatoes control group. However, there were eight deaths from heart disease among the Prudent Diet group, and none among those who ate meat three times a day. (Dr. Jolliffe the lead author died in 1966 from a vascular thrombosis.)

In 1987, Anderson, Castelli, and Levy, published their study: "Cholesterol and Mortality: 30 Years of Follow-up from the Framingham Study" in the Journal of the American Medical Association. The Framingham study is a long-term study that looked at serum cholesterol levels in 1,959 men and 2,415 women from 1951 to 1955. The individuals were between 31 – 65 years and free of cardiovascular disease. The authors found that after age 50 years of age, there is no increased overall mortality with either high or low serum cholesterol levels.

Harcombe *et al.* conducted a systemic review

and meta-analysis of reports, published prior to 1983, which examined the relationship between dietary fat, serum cholesterol and the development of heart disease that may have been used to support the dietary fat guidelines of 1977 and 1983. The dietary fat guidelines were released by the US (1977) and UK (1983) governments to significantly reduce saturated fat consumption. Shockingly, the authors concluded that evidence from randomized controlled trials **did not** support the recommendations introduced in the dietary fat guidelines! They concluded that "dietary recommendations were introduced for 220 million US and 56 million UK citizens by 1983, in the absence of supporting evidence from RCTs" (Random Controlled Trials). Data from six (6) clinical studies of men with coronary heart-disease had blood-cholesterol lower than the expected values!

The *Honolulu Heart Program* looked at cholesterol concentrations in 3,572 Japanese/American men (aged 71–93 years). They compared changes in cholesterol levels over 20 years to all-cause mortality. Mean cholesterol fell significantly with increasing age, and those individuals with low cholesterol had an increase in the number of deaths. This casts doubt on the recommendation of lowering cholesterol levels, especially in the elderly.

Research published in March 1993 showed that heart disease worsened in those who switched from butter to polyunsaturated-rich margarine. The study compared 85,000 women who ate polyunsaturated margarine, to those who did not consume margarine.

Those who ate four (4) or more teaspoons of polyunsaturated margarine a day had a sixty-six (66%) percent *increased* risk of coronary heart disease (CHD). A similar review of men in the *Framingham Study* published in 1995 also found that six (6) teaspoons a day increased risk by nearly a third. The authors conclude: "Intake of margarine may predispose to development of CHD in men".

In 1996, an article was published in the Israel Journal of Medical Science titled: *Diet and disease--the Israeli paradox: possible dangers of a high omega-6 polyunsaturated fatty acid diet*. The authors state that "Israel has one of the highest dietary polyunsaturated/saturated fat ratios in the world; the consumption of omega-6 polyunsaturated fatty acids (PUFA) is about 8% higher than in the USA, and 10-12% higher than in most European countries." They conclude that "despite such national habits, there is paradoxically a high prevalence of cardiovascular diseases, hypertension, non-insulin-dependent diabetes mellitus and obesity; all diseases that are associated with hyperinsulinemia (HI) and insulin resistance (IR), and grouped together as the insulin resistance syndrome or syndrome X. There is also an increased cancer incidence and mortality rate, especially in women, compared with western countries. Studies suggest that high omega-6 linoleic acid consumption might aggravate HI and IR, in addition to being a substrate for lipid peroxidation and free radical formation. Thus, rather than being beneficial, high omega-6 PUFA diets may have some long-term side effects, within the cluster of hyperinsulinemia, atherosclerosis and tumorigenesis."

It has been known since 1994 that intake of poly-unsaturated fats affects the fatty-acid content of aortic plaques. Felton *et al.* compared the fatty-acid composition of aortic plaques with that of post-mortem serum and adipose tissue. They found a positive association between serum and adipose omega-3, omega-6 polyunsaturated fatty acids as well as monounsaturated fatty acids, with plaque formation. No associations were found with saturated fatty acids. These findings imply a direct influence of dietary polyunsaturated fatty acids on aortic plaque formation.

A study in postmenopausal women by Mozaffarian and colleagues found that those women with a higher saturated fat intake had less coronary atherosclerosis progression while polyunsaturated fatty acid (PUFA) intake was associated with worsening in the diameter of the coronary artery. They found for each 5% increase in energy intake from PUFA, there was a 0.17 mm greater decline in minimal coronary artery diameter and a 5.8% greater progression in mean percentage stricture. The intake of PUFA was also associated with increased atherosclerosis progression when replacing saturated fat Moreover, a greater intake of saturated fat was not associated with adverse cardiovascular outcomes

An article in the journal *Annals of Internal Medicine*, published in 2003 identified 72 studies: 45 cohort studies and 27 randomized controlled trials looking at the association between dietary fatty acid intake and coronary disease. The 32 cohort studies included 530,525 people. When comparing the top third to those in the bottom third of dietary fatty acid intake, only trans fatty acid intake was significantly associated with a risk of coronary disease. This comprehensive review found no evidence that saturated fat increases the risk of coronary disease, or that polyunsaturated fats have a cardio protective effect, in contrast to current recommendations! Since then, numerous meta-analyses of prospective epidemiologic studies have concluded the same; that there is no significant evidence for concluding that dietary saturated fat is associated with an increased risk of coronary heart disease or cardiovascular disease.

Even the American Heart Association has backed away from their long-held recommendation of reducing dietary cholesterol. "As anticipated, the panel did not include a recommendation for dietary cholesterol, agreeing with an *American Heart Association/American College of Cardiology* report that concluded "there isn't scientific evidence to show it reduces the artery-clogging LDL cholesterol in the blood". In the *2010 Dietary Guidelines*, Americans were told to limit dietary cholesterol to 300 mg a day.

Galvao *et al.*, in 2012 compared a standard low-fat diet to high-fat diets enriched with either saturated fat (palmitate and stearate) or PUFA (linoleic and α-linolenic acids) in hamsters with genetic cardiomyopathy. Their results show that a high intake of saturated fat improves survival in heart failure compared with a high PUFA diet or low-fat diet. They also found an increase in mitochondrial permeability in the PUFA group. This confirmed the work of Galvao *et al.* from a previous year, showing that heart failure hamsters fed a diet high in saturated fat showed increased survival compared with hamsters fed a diet high in PUFA or the control standard diet.

In 2013, the results of the Sydney Diet Heart Study were published. The study, titled: *Use of Dietary Linoleic Acid for Secondary Prevention of Coronary Heart Disease and Death*, looked at the effectiveness of replacing dietary saturated fat with omega 6 linoleic acid, for the secondary prevention of coronary heart disease and death. Participants were 458 men aged 30-59 years with a recent coronary event. They replaced dietary saturated fats with omega-6 linoleic acid (from safflower oil and safflower oil polyunsaturated margarine). Controls received no specific dietary instruction or study foods. Substituting dietary linoleic acid in place of saturated fats increased the rate of death from all causes, coronary heart disease, and cardiovascular disease. An up dated meta-analysis of linoleic acid intervention trials showed no evidence of cardiovascular benefit.

Despite the overwhelming evidence to the contrary, the American College of Cardiology and American Heart Association continued to demonize saturated fats. Their 2013 guidelines on lifestyle management to reduce CVD risk omitted a target for total dietary fat but did recommend a goal of 5%-6% of calories from saturated fat.

The basis for their argument is the observation that polyunsaturated fats decrease levels of serum LDL-cholesterol, thereby reducing cardiovascular disease. Yet, this hypothesis is easily proven false. In a meta-analysis of over 60 trials, higher intakes of saturated fat were, as expected, associated with an increase in LDL-cholesterol levels. However, there was an increase in high-density lipoprotein cholesterol (HDL-C) as well, coupled with a decrease in triglyceride levels, for a net neutral effect on the ratio of total cholesterol to HDL cholesterol. Although saturated fats increase LDL-C, they reduce the LDL particle number. Total LDL particle number is considered a stronger indicator of CV risk than traditional cholesterol measures.

These studies suggest that a diet containing saturated fats is either neutral, or prolongs life compared with a diet high in polyunsaturated fat. Not only is there a lack of survival benefit with the high PUFA diet, but the high PUFA diet is associated with a 75% increase in plasma free fatty acids. Clinical studies in the 1960s found an association between elevated free fatty acids and ventricular arrhythmias. It was later shown that plasma fatty acid concentration is a strong predictor of sudden cardiac death. While it is possible that the elevation in free fatty acids triggers arrhythmias, there is further evidence that PUFA's are directly involved with the pathogenesis of atherosclerosis.

2. What is Cholesterol?

To better understand atherosclerosis, and the role polyunsaturated acid play in the development of heart disease, we need to have a basic understanding of the mechanisms involved. I often hear about the artery clogging effects of fats. Even the American Heart Association mentions "artery-clogging LDL cholesterol" in their literature. These are frequent seen in articles on atherosclerosis and usually followed with a discussion on the "good fats (polyunsaturated vegetable oil) and the "bad fats" (saturated fats). It is unfortunate that the scientific method has failed us and marketing strategies prevail over our understanding of the pathogenesis of this disease.

Cholesterol is a lipid molecule and is manufactured by all animal cells. It is a major structural molecule in cell walls, as well as a precursor for the biosynthesis of steroid hormones, bile acids, and vitamin D. Cholesterol is only slightly soluble in water. So, to enable cholesterol transport in the blood, cholesterol must be transported inside vesicles called lipoproteins.

There are several types of lipoproteins found in the blood. In order of increasing density, they are chylomicrons, very-low-density lipoprotein (VLDL), low-density lipoprotein (LDL), intermediate-density lipoprotein (IDL), and high-density lipoprotein (HDL). So, when a physician orders a fractionated cholesterol panel, the results are just a profile of the different lipoproteins.

LDL particles are the major blood cholesterol carriers. Each one contains approximately 1,500 molecules of cholesterol. The LDL cholesterol particle is a spherical globule with a lipoprotein - apo B embedded in its matrix. The HDL particle is similar to the LDL lipoprotein except for the presence of apo A in its matrix (Figure 4).

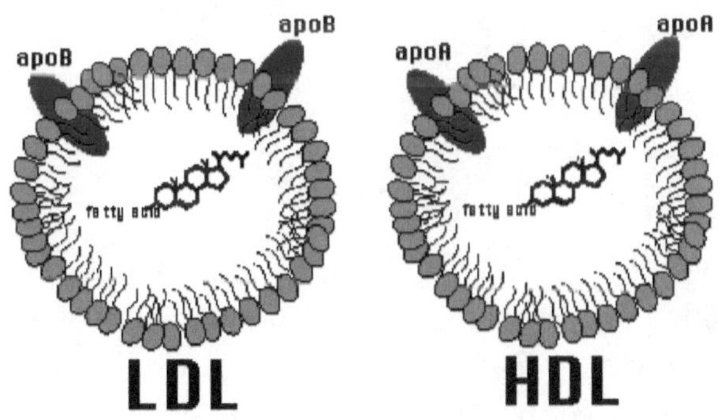

Figure 4: LDL and HDL lipoproteins. The LDL and HDL cholesterol particle are spherical globule with a lipoprotein - apo B is embedded in the matrix of the LDL particle.

Nature has developed this elegant means of transporting cholesterol around the body. As a cell senses the need for cholesterol, it produces apo B protein receptors on its cell membrane. The Apo B binds to the receptor protein and the LDL particle is released into the cell cytoplasm (Figure 5).

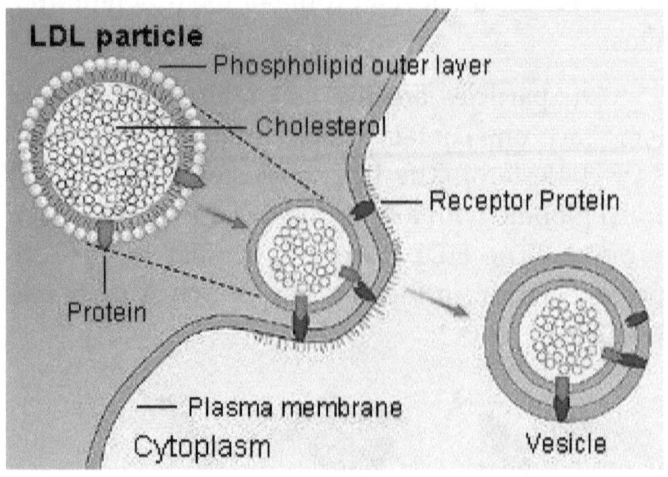

Figure 5: The LDL particle binds to Apo-B receptors on the cell membrane thereby releasing cholesterol into the cell.

The reverse is true if a cell has too much cholesterol. The HDL particle transports excess cholesterol to the liver where it is recycled (Figure 6). Cholesterol levels are tightly controlled and individual levels are "set" due to that person's genetic predisposition. In other words, as you consume more cholesterol, the liver reduces the amount manufactured, as well as the corollary, the less you consume, the more is produced. Overall, 90% of cholesterol is synthesized in the liver so dietary cholesterol impact is negligible.

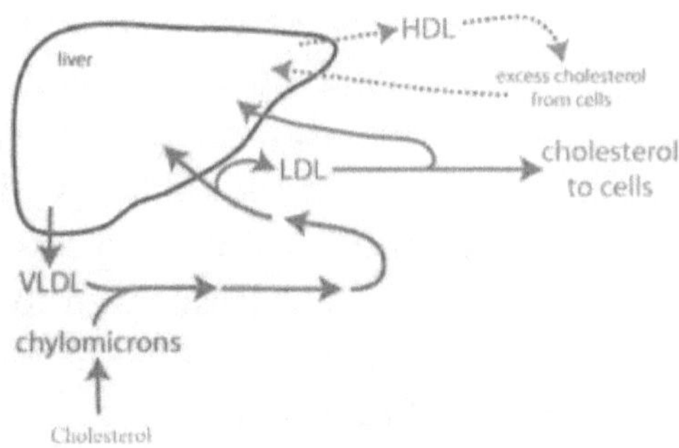

Figure 6: lipoproteins transport cholesterol to cells. Excess cholesterol is removed by HDL where it is returned to the liver for recycling. Dietary cholesterol is transported via chylomicrons either to the liver or eventually to LDL particles.

Familial hypercholesterolemia (High cholesterol **caused by a specific genetic defect**) is due to a defect in the LDL receptor that prevents the clearance of LDL particles from the circulation.

Atherosclerosis

Investigators began to notice in the 1980's that half of those who suffer coronary heart disease had LDL-cholesterol levels with-in normal limits. In the *Women's Health Study*, 46% of first cardiovascular events occurred in women with LDL cholesterol levels less than 130 mg/dL, the "desirable" target for primary prevention set by the *National Cholesterol Education Program* (NCEP). Castelli published a series of articles noting that more than 75 percent of patients with an acute coronary syndrome or a myocardial infarction had normal plasma values of cholesterol, LDL cholesterol and/or HDL cholesterol.

The protective effects of statins against cardiovascular disease as seen in the *Scandinavian Simvastatin Survival Study Group* did not stand up to challenges from other clinical studies. As with many studies showing decreases in plasma LDL cholesterol with statin administration, the protection against cardiovascular disease was simply not there. At least seven follow-on studies suggest that LDL-cholesterol blood level is unlikely to be an important causal factor for cardiovascular disease.

The clinical failure of the cholesterol lowering drug Vytorin in the ENHANCE Trial (*The Effect of Combination Ezetimibe and High-Dose Simvastatin vs. Simvastatin Alone on the Atherosclerotic Process in Patients with Heterozygous Familial Hypercholesterolemia*) is prompting a reexamination of the rational for using statins to treat atherosclerosis. Statins are sold by numerous pharmaceutical companies. Lovastatin (Mevacor) and simvastatin (Zocor); rosuvastatin (Crestor); pravastatin (Pravachol); Fluvastatin (Lescol); and atorvastatin (Lipitor). Vytorin is a formulation that combines simvastatin with a non-statin cholesterol absorption blocker, ezetimibe (Zetia).

The ENHANCE trial showed a significant decrease in low-density lipoprotein cholesterol (LDL-C) levels over the two years of the study as expected. However, the intima-media thickness (IMT) in the arteries increased in both groups, but was significantly greater in the Vytorin group than in the simvastatin group! IMT is considered to be an important marker of atherosclerosis and a strong predictor of future myocardial infarction. In other words, the reduction in cholesterol levels did not make a difference in preventing atherosclerosis. However, the combined effect of two cholesterol agents accelerated atherosclerosis! The trial was eventually published in *New England Journal of Medicine* in April, 2008 after some delay.

The ENHANCE trial simply confirmed the findings that Abramson and Wright published in 2007. They conducted a meta-analysis of eight randomized controlled trials and concluded (1) total mortality is not reduced with statin therapy, (2) serious adverse events were not reduced either, and (3) the absolute frequency of cardiovascular events was reduced by only 1.5%! In other words, you would have to treat 67 patients with statins over a 5-year period for one patient to benefit (a 98.5% failure rate).

To be fair, not all statins are equal in their ability to reduce LDL-cholesterol. So, let's look at CRESTOR (rosuvastatin calcium) which is widely regarded to be one of the most potent statins. According to the FDA approved labeling, Crestor lowers LDL-cholesterol by an average of 55% after 12 weeks of dosing at 20mg per day.

As justification of approval, the label references the JUPITER study (*In the Justification for the Use of Statins in Primary Prevention: An Intervention Trial Evaluating Rosuvastatin*). "The effect of CRESTOR (rosuvastatin calcium) on the occurrence of major cardiovascular (CV) disease events was assessed in 17,802 men ($\geq$ 50 years) and women ($\geq$ 60 years) who had no clinically evident cardiovascular disease ". Study participants had a median baseline LDL-C of 108 mg/dL. Study participants were randomly assigned to placebo (n=8,901) or rosuvastatin 20 mg once daily (n=8,901) and were followed for a mean duration of 2 years. Rosuvastatin reduced the risk of major CV events with an absolute risk reduction of just 1.2%!

In other words, the absolute risk reduction of having a major cardiovascular event after taking Crestor for two years is in line with the meta-analysis of the other statin trials. This is hardly a ringing endorsement of the cholesterol hypothesis.

When examining the major statin trials, and looking across various strengths of statin drugs, what becomes apparent is these cholesterol lowering drugs have not demonstrated an all-cause mortality benefit for patients. And yet they continue to be prescribed at an increasing rate despite a range of serious harmful effects.

In a large clinical study involving over 10,000 participants who were randomly assigned to two groups for comparison; those using very high dose Lipitor (80mg) achieved markedly lower LDL-C levels compared to those using a much lower dose of Pravastatin (10mg). Yet, there were 26 fewer deaths in the lower dose group. Unexpectedly, the total number of deaths from causes other than cardiac events was greater in the high dose group, exceeding those in the low dose group by 31. The lack of benefit was not loss on the *New England Journal of Medicine* who stated in their editorial that *"further assurances as to the safety of this approach was needed"* (NEJM 2005).

In 2012. H. Petursson *et al.*, examined cholesterol levels used in mortality risk algorithms in clinical guidelines based on ten years of prospective data from the *Norwegian HUNT 2* study. The study population comprised 52,087 Norwegians, aged 20–74, who participated in the Nord-Trøndelag Health Study (HUNT 2) from 1995–1997, and were followed-up on cause-specific mortality for 10 years (510,97 person-years in total). The authors concluded that "public health recommendations regarding the 'dangers' of cholesterol should be revised. This is especially true for women, for whom moderately elevated cholesterol (by current standards) may prove to be not only harmless but even beneficial."

K. Anderson *et al.*, examined the relationship of cholesterol and mortality based on 30 Years of follow-up from the *Framingham Study*. From 1951 to 1955 serum cholesterol levels were measured in 1,959 men and 2,415 women aged between 31 and 65 years who were free of cardiovascular disease (CVD) and cancer. They found that under age 50 years, cholesterol levels are directly related with 30-year overall and CVD mortality. However, after age 50 years there is no increased overall mortality with either high or low serum cholesterol levels!

In 2012, Saremi *et al.*, published an association with frequent statin use and an accelerated progression of coronary artery calcification in a study of 197 diabetic patients without previous coronary artery disease. The frequent statin users had significantly lower, and nearly optimal, LDL-cholesterol levels. Yet, despite the lowering of cholesterol levels, the use of statins was associated with an acceleration of calcific atherosclerosis.

Other randomized controlled trials in largely nondiabetic populations, with no previous coronary artery disease, have demonstrated that statin drugs accelerate the progression of coronary artery calcification, as well, as abdominal aortic artery calcification. These results were confirmed by R. Nakazat *et al.*, in 2012, analyzing statins use and coronary artery plaque composition based on results from the *International Multicenter CONFIRM Registry*. The authors identified 6,673 individuals (2,413 on statin therapy and 4,260 not on statin therapy) with no known CAD, and with available statin use status. They studied the relationship between statin use and the presence and extent of specific plaque composition types, which was graded as non-calcified (NCP), mixed (MP), or calcified (CP) plaque. Compared to the individuals not taking statins, those taking statins had a <u>higher</u> prevalence of risk factors and obstructive CAD leading the authors to conclude that statin use is associated with an increased prevalence and extent of coronary plaques possessing calcium.

Despite the published findings of lack of benefit with cholesterol lowering drugs, several pharmaceutical companies set out to develop a new class of cholesterol lowering drugs called *CEPT inhibitors*. A CETP inhibitor inhibits the cholesteryl ester transfer protein (CETP), and are designed to substantially increases HDL-cholesterol, and reverse cholesterol transport.

The results of the *Investigation of Lipid Level Management to Understand its Impact in Atherosclerotic Events* (ILLUMINATE) trial were published in *The New England Journal of Medicine* in 2007. The trial involved 15,067 patients (mean age 61 years) with coronary heart disease (CHD), or at risk for CHD (type 2 diabetes). Patients underwent a run-in period of 4-10 weeks during which they received lifestyle counseling, with or without atorvastatin (statin), to achieve a low-density lipoprotein cholesterol (LDL-C) goal of <100 mg/dL. Patients who achieved that target at the end of the run-in period were randomized to atorvastatin at the dose established during run-in, plus torcetrapib 60 mg (CETP inhibitor), or placebo. The trial was planned to run for 4.5 years.

At 12 months, patients who received torcetrapib showed an unprecedented panel of cholesterol results, including:

- Mean increase of 72.1% in HDL-cholesterol;
- Mean decrease of 24.9% in LDL-cholesterol; and
- Small mean decrease of 9% in triglycerides compared with baseline.

These lipid effects were consistent with those in previous studies. The primary endpoint of the trial was a composite of first major cardiovascular event, defined as coronary heart disease (CHD) death, nonfatal myocardial infarction (MI), stroke, or hospitalization for unstable angina. At termination, the torcetrapib group showed a 25% increased risk over the groups that received atorvastatin alone.

If the deposition of cholesterol in the plaques is not due to LDL, then some altered form of lipoprotein must be responsible. It seems that only a fraction of the LDL universe is atherogenic, with the majority of circulating LDL not contributing to coronary disease. Therefore, the reduction of total LDL-cholesterol as a target for hypolipidemic treatment for prevention of atherosclerosis is chasing after the wrong blood marker.

Particularly atherogenic forms of LDL include small, dense LDL particles and oxidized LDL. The small LDL particles are manufactured in the liver in response to fructose in the diet. Studies have shown that fructose (a sugar found in fruit) ingestion is associated with a decrease of LDL particle size and an increase in its density. This effect is not limited to fructose either, since sucrose (table sugar) breaks down to glucose and fructose when ingested. High-carbohydrate diets therefore reduce plasma LDL cholesterol, but also provokes the appearance of an atherogenic lipoprotein profile, characterized by high plasma triglycerides, small dense LDL particles, and reduced HDL cholesterol.

3. The Endothelium

The endothelium is the inner cell lining of all blood vessels and lymphatics in the body. Early descriptions of the cardiovascular system by the Ancient Greeks, depicted the veins and arteries as completely separate systems They observed arteries as deeply situated, thick, pulsating vessels containing red blood, and veins as superficial, distended, thin walled, non-pulsating vessels carrying blue blood.

Blood was not seen to circulate, but rather to ebb and flow in these two systems of blood vessels. This view of the cardiovascular system prevailed until William Harvey's discovery of blood circulation in 1628. The following 200 years would witness an intense debate about the true nature of capillaries; did they have a wall or, as many believed, were simply tunnels drilled into the tissue It wasn't until much later with the introduction of silver nitrate staining that the presence of a cellular lining (or capillary wall) was realized.

The term endothelium was first described in 1865 to distinguish the inner lining of blood vessels from the epithelial layers. This led to astounding increase in the number of publications related to endothelial cells and the endothelium, as well as advances in our understanding of this cell type.

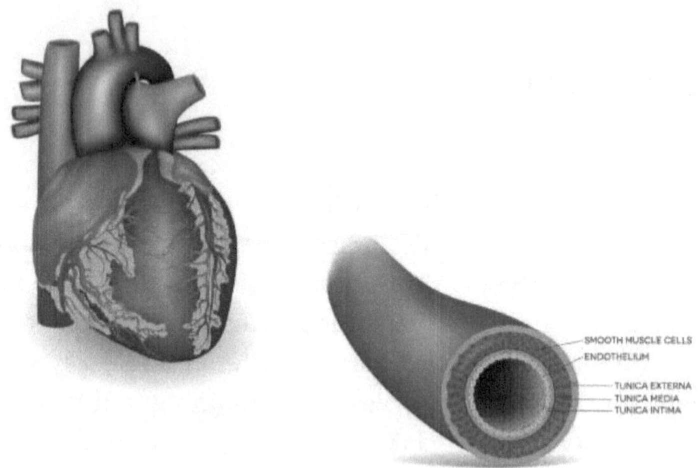

Figure 7: The endothelium is a single layer of cells that line the inner surface of all blood and lymphatic vessels, forming an interface between circulating blood or lymph.

The endothelium is a single layer of cells that line the inner surface of all blood and lymphatic vessels. Physiologically, it forms an interface between circulating blood or lymph in the vessel lumen forming a barrier between vessels and tissue.

Oxidized LDL (ox-LDL) is chemotactic for monocytes (Chemotaxis is the movement of a cell in response to a chemical stimulus). In other words, monocytes are attracted to the ox-LDL particle through scavenger receptors binding on the monocyte. Following binding to the ox-LDL particle, monocytes transform themselves into macrophages. Ox-LDL binds with high affinity to the scavenger receptors on the macrophage plasma membrane, which leads to the internalization of the ox-LDL and lead to its degradation (Figure 8).

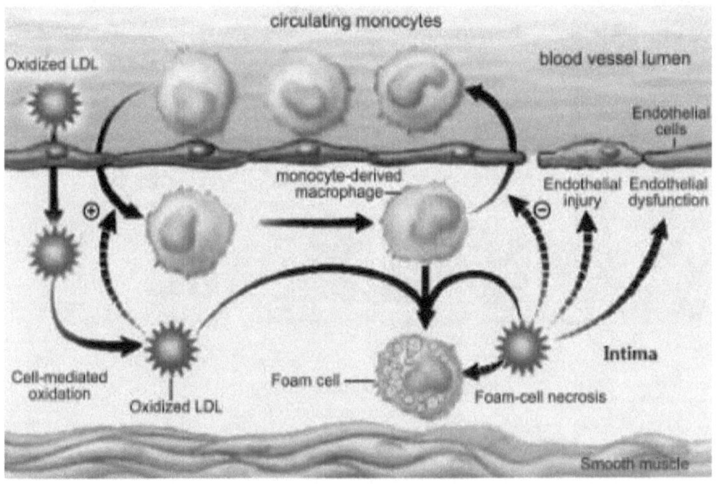

Figure 8: Oxidized cholesterol triggers the migration of monocyte/macrophage which engulf the LDL particle. The cholesterol engorged macrophage transform into foam cells which eventually die forming the plaque seen in atherosclerosis.

The macrophage engulfs the ox-LDL particle eventually becoming a "Foam cell". The conversion of monocyte-to-macrophage differentiation is specific to ox-LDL, and not native LDL. It is also dependent on the extent of LDL oxidation, and requires ox-LDL internalization by the cells. The lipid-laden "foam cells" observed in early atherosclerotic lesions appear to be monocyte/macrophages that have taken up cholesterol in the intimal space. Malondialdehyde, from peroxidized polyunsaturated fatty acids, induces avid uptake of cholesterol by the scavenger receptor of human monocyte-macrophages!

Eventually, the burst of the atherosclerotic plaque due to high blood pressure results in the blockage of the artery. Atherosclerosis develops quietly though for many years before clinical manifestation are revealed.

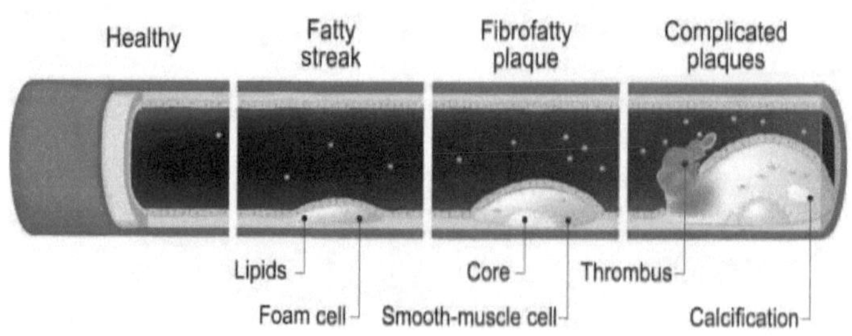

Figure 9: Stages of atherosclerosis development.

The knowledge that LDL-cholesterol is extremely susceptible to oxidative damage has been known for some time. To date, there are over 10,000 journal articles on oxidized LDL. It is now clear from the large volume of literature, that oxidized LDL cholesterol is a critical factor in the development of atherosclerosis.

But what is the initiating event which begins the process of atherosclerosis? The earliest detectable changes in the course of an atherosclerotic lesion are manifested in lesion-prone areas of the arterial vasculature. Therefore, Endothelial cell dysfunction (ECD) is where we begin.

Endothelial dysfunction is characterized by a reduction of the availability of vasodilators, in particular, nitric oxide (NO). Vasodilators are chemical messengers that signal the smooth muscles of the arteries to relax. This imbalance leads to an impairment of endothelium-dependent vasodilation. In addition, endothelial dysfunction is also characterized by a proinflammatory, proliferative, and pro-coagulatory environment that favors the development of atherogenesis.

Those known risk factors that are related to atherosclerosis and cardiovascular death, are also associated with endothelial dysfunction. These risk factors, which include hyperlipidemia, hypertension, diabetes, and smoking are also associated with overproduction of reactive oxygen species and increased oxidative stress. Reactive oxygen species (ROS) interact with nitric oxide, which reduces the bioavailability of NO and thereby promotes cellular damage. Thus, increased oxidative stress is considered a major mechanism involved in the pathogenesis of endothelial dysfunction.

It is widely recognized that linoleic acid (LA), an omega-6 polyunsaturated fatty acid, found in plant oils increases the expression of adhesion molecules and disrupts endothelial cell function. Adhesion molecules are cell surface proteins that facilitates the interaction between cells. Linoleic acid enhances the expression of adhesion molecules in endothelial cells and promotes inflammatory cell migration, resulting in the development of endothelial dysfunction.

Linoleic acid is the major polyunsaturated fatty acid found in common vegetable oils. Linoleic acid is also known to elicit an inflammatory response, and is proatherogenic by causing arterial smooth muscle cell proliferation. Furthermore, there is evidence that Linoleic acid, is atherogenic by directly causing endothelial injury. Omega-6 PUFAs, such as Linoleic acid and arachidonic acid, are able to release calcium from internal stores and thereby induce calcium entry into the cells. A change in intracellular calcium is an early and critical event in the development of cytotoxicity, causing the ultimate loss of endothelial cell viability

Omega-6 fats modulate endothelial cell calcium which in turn decreases the production of endothelial factors such as NO, which, under oxidative stress, can lead to the formation of peroxynitrites, a vascular toxin. Peroxynitrite, is formed by the reaction between NO and superoxide anion. Peroxynitrite can react with a wide range of biomolecules to result in lipid peroxidation, causing damage to cellular constituents including proteins, DNA, and lipids. Therefore, the formation of peroxynitrite may result in the loss of many of the beneficial effects of NO, including vasodilation.

Peroxisome proliferator-activated receptors (PPARα, β, γ) are factors that regulate various cellular processes including fat and glucose control Both PPARα and PPARγ are found in vascular cells including endothelial cells, smooth muscle cells, as well as in monocyte and macrophages cells. Activators of PPARs have beneficial effects against atherosclerosis by regulating the anti-inflammatory pathways in vascular cells. Atherogenic omega-6 lipids, such as linoleic acid and its oxidized forms, 13-hydroperoxy octadecadienoic acid (13-HODE) and 13-hydroxyoctadecadienoic acid (13-HODE) bind directly to both PPARα and PPARγ, thereby altering their activity.

<u>Endothelial Microparticles</u>

Perhaps the most convincing bit of evidence for omega-6 polyunsaturated fats causing endothelial toxicity is the production of endothelial microparticles. Circulating numbers of endothelial microparticles (EMP) are an index of endothelial injury and dysfunction. Most importantly, oxidative stress, is responsible for EMP release causing endothelial cells to undergo functional changes, eventually leading to the pathology of atherosclerosis.

As endothelial cells undergo injury, they release endothelial microparticles (EMP) which can be measured as an index of endothelial injury and dysfunction. Microparticles are small vesicles that are released from cells through plasma membrane budding, leading to the formation of membrane blebs (figure 10).

Acute endothelial injury, such as that induced by secondhand smoke, rapidly compromises endothelial function and increases circulating EMP in healthy subjects. Therefore, endothelial microparticles are a useful marker for endothelial injury.

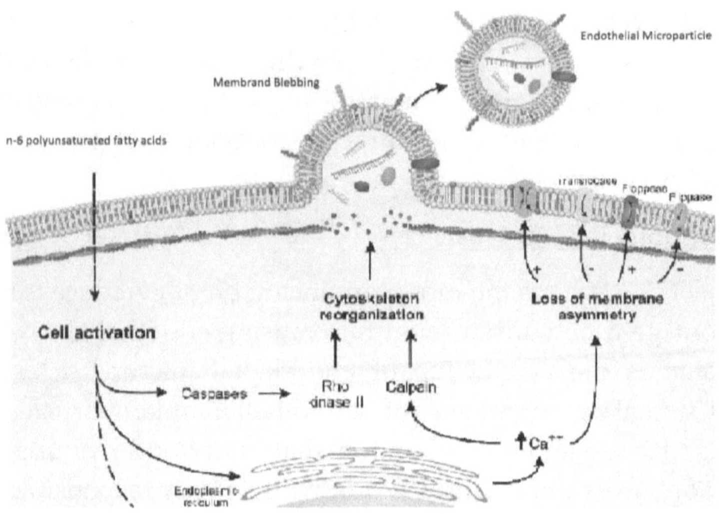

Figure 10: Endothelial microparticles. N-6 polyunsaturated fats activate the cell creating membrane blebbing,

Researches have demonstrated the key role of EMPs in the growth, division, and maturation of endothelial precursor cells – those cells that eventually mature to form endothelial cells. These cells are important for blood vessel regeneration suggesting a potential preservative role in response to vascular regeneration, restoration, and protection. Therefore, endothelial microparticles are critical part of the progression of unstable atherosclerotic plaques.

4. The Oxidized Lipid Hypothesis

As mentioned previously, atherosclerosis begins with injury to the endothelial cells lining medium and large arteries. There is significant evidence that suggests exposure to dietary omega-6 polyunsaturated fatty acids can directly affect endothelial cell metabolism. Significant amounts of data have been accumulated to show that linoleic acid can induce discernable injury to endothelial cells in blood vessels. An internet search using the search term "linoleic acid and endothelial dysfunction" will yield over 2,390,000 hits! Using the same parameters, but substituting arachidonic acid, will yield over 737,000 hits. This vast amount of data leads to one conclusion: these *n-6* fatty acids damage the endothelial walls of arteries.

The effects of n-6 fatty acids on endothelial cells are numerous. There is a significant increase in adhesion of monocytes to the endothelial monolayer in the presence of n-6 fatty acids. These unsaturated fats are involved in oxidative stress, cellular dysfunction, mitochondrial dysfunction, inflammation, and apoptosis (cell death). So, from this we can postulate that n-6 fatty acids can induce the first step in atherosclerosis – endothelial injury.

Endothelial microparticles increase significantly following fatty fast-food meals that are rich in poly-saturated fatty acids as well as their lipid oxidation products. Sutherland (*et al.* 2010) took twenty-two healthy subjects and fed them meals either rich in cream, unheated sunflower oil, or heated sunflower oil, then observed them for release of microparticles at 1 and 3 hours post meal. They found that ingestion of meals rich in n-6 polyunsaturated vegetable oil, irre-spective of whether it has been mildly thermally oxi-dized, significantly increased the number of EMP, whereas the group receiving saturated fats had no ef-fect. The subjects who ate the polyunsaturated oil had a 20% increase in endothelial microparticles! They con-cluded that n-6 polyunsaturated fats may acutely alter the state of the vascular endothelium, resulting in in-creased shedding of EMP.

We know that atherosclerosis is not the result of the uptake of native LDL, which itself is incapable of causing cholesterol accumulation in mono-cyte/macrophages, but instead is due to the uptake of one or more oxidized forms of LDL. What is the source of this modified LDL? This is the subject of some de-bate. But it is clear that diet plays a significant role; es-pecially with linoleic acid oxidation products.

When rabbits are fed a diet rich in oxidized li-pid, there is a 100% increase in fatty streak lesions in the aorta and a >100% increase in total cholesterol in the pulmonary artery. Additionally, when rats are fed oxidized corn oil, there is a significantly increased aortic wall thickness after just six months of dietary feeding.

If we look at the composition of the atherosclerotic plaque for clues, we find high levels of hydroxyoctadecanoic acids (derived from linoleic acid), 15-hydroxyeicosatetranoic acid (derived from arachidonic acid), and 11-HETE (derived from arachidonic acid) in all atherosclerotic plaques. Low levels of 9-oxo-octadecanoic acid (from linoleic acid), and 13-oxoODE from linoleic acid) are also present. What is important to note from these observations is the compounds found in the plaques are the oxidation products of linoleic and arachidonic acid, both omega-6 polyunsaturated fatty acids found in vegetable oils.

An article in the *Lancet* in 1994 looked at dietary polyunsaturated fatty acid and composition of human aortic plaques. It compared the fatty acid composition of post-mortem blood samples to the fatty acid composition of aortic plaques and adipose tissue (adipose tissue, or body fat reflects the dietary intake of fatty acids). While there were no associations with saturated fatty acids, they did conclude that there is "a direct influence of dietary polyunsaturated fatty acids on aortic plaque formation and suggest that current trends favoring increased intake of polyunsaturated fatty acids should be reconsidered."

Another study examined 50 subjects with coronary artery disease (defined as >50% narrowing in one or more major coronary vessels), and 54 without coronary artery disease, looking at systemic levels of specific fatty acid oxidation products. They found 9-HETE and F(2)-isoprostanes, were significantly elevated in patients with coronary artery disease. Both are oxidation products of arachidonic acid, again supporting the hypothesis that *n-6* polyunsaturated fatty acids are responsible for plaque formation in coronary artery disease.

Studies going back to 1997 show that the oxidation products in atherosclerotic plaques are products of linoleic and arachidonic acid, both polyunsaturated fats. Gniwotta *et al.*, in 1997 concluded the "data show that human atherosclerotic lesions contain increased amounts of hydroxyl-linoleic acid isomers and isoprostanes when compared with non-atherosclerotic vessel wall and suggest a link between local lipid peroxidation and progression of atherosclerosis."

Waddington *et al.*, in 2003, published an article describing presence of fatty acid oxidation products in histological samples of atherosclerosis plaque. They found, as have others, that arachidonic acid oxidation products were significantly higher in those subjects who also had coronary artery disease.

From this evidence one can deduce that linoleic acid is a precursor to the oxidized linoleic metabolites found in atherosclerotic plaques. Humans cannot synthesize linoleic acid, so our diet is the sole source. These linoleic acid stores in visceral fat, in turn, serve as the substrate for endogenous oxidized linoleic metabolites, although oxidized linoleic metabolites are obtained via the diet as well. Studies have shown that lowering dietary linoleic acid from 6.7% to 2.4% of calories can significantly lower oxidized linoleic metabolites.

Studies have also demonstrated that oxidized polyunsaturated fatty acid products, including oxidized linoleic acid, are absorbed by the small intestine and incorporated into chylomicrons. Increased peroxide levels are seen in chylomicrons, VLDL, and LDL lipoproteins. Therefore, oxidized linoleic acid products are efficiently incorporated into the LDL particle leading to ox-LDL. The oxidation of lipoproteins does not just result in the creation of a single molecular species, but a variety of oxidation products. One specific target of LDL oxidation that is of particular importance is the Apo B lipoprotein on the LDL particle. As the LDL-particle undergoes oxidation, the products of lipid peroxidation (such as HNE or other aldehyde products), bind to the lysine residues on Apo B. This results in the modification of the Apo B molecule, which induces a recognition by the scavenger receptor on tissue macrophages.

5. Epidemiological Evidence

If LDL-cholesterol levels were the cause of atherosclerosis, then we would expect the incidence of coronary artery disease to be similar across different geographies and populations. However, this is not the

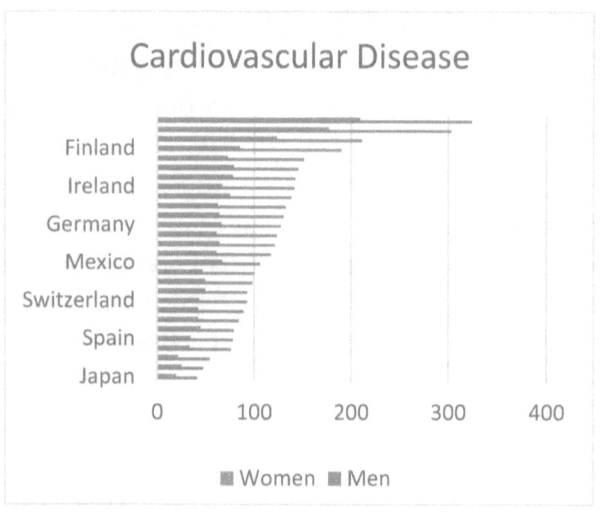

Figure 11: Incidence of cardiovascular disease age-standardized rates per 100,000 of the population.

case. As you can see in figure 11, the incidence of cardiovascular disease in the United States is significantly higher than other countries, suggesting that dietary factors are in play.

The age adjusted incidence of cardiovascular disease in the United State is 145 cases per 100,000 people. Compare this rate to Japan, France, or Korea whose rates are 66% lower than the US rate for cardiovascular disease, and you must conclude that some other factor is in play. One obvious difference is diet.

A dietary aspect we should be able to dismiss is the hypothesis that consumption of saturated fat is somehow correlated to cardiovascular disease. Despite recommendations to reduce the amount of saturated fat in the diet, there is no correlation between saturated fat and deaths due to coronary heart disease when com-paring different geographies, as shown in figure 12. In fact, France has the highest consumption of satu-

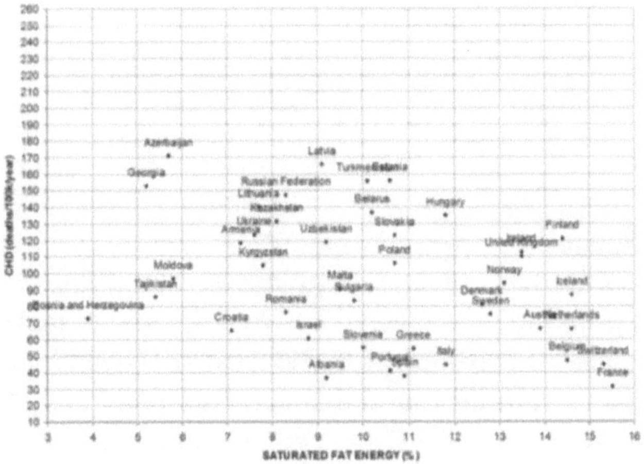

Figure 12: Percent of saturated fat energy (%) vs coronary heart disease deaths/100,000/year) in European men 1998.

rated fat and the lowest rate of heart disease! Given what we have discussed previously on saturated fat, it does not appear saturated fats have an impact on deaths due to coronary heart disease.

However, if we look at arachidonic acid content of adipose tissue in across different countries, and compare this to heart disease mortality, we see a different picture, and a clear correlation with arachidonic acid (20:4 polyunsaturated fat) and cardiac mortality (figure 13).

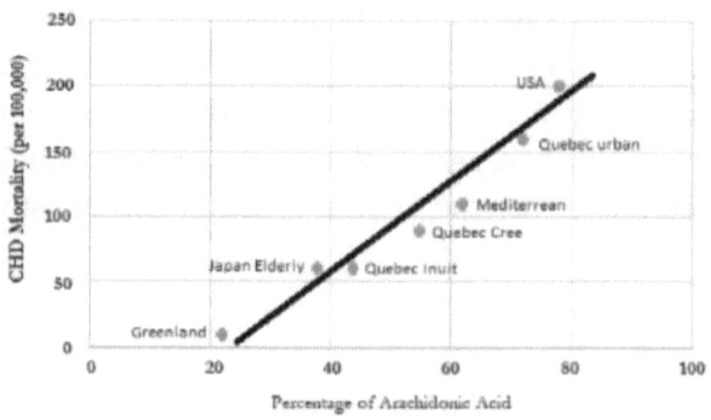

Figure 13: Mortality rates due to heart disease and tissue arachidonic acid.

Let's next look at populations that have not been exposed to seed oils, which are very few in number. A study published in the journal of *Tropical and Geographical Medicine* found that coronary heart disease is virtually unknown in the Vedda population of Sri Lanka. The Vedda communities in the South Eastern jungles of Sri Lanka consume a diet of fruits, yams, coconuts, and hunting wild game. The majority of dietary fat in the traditional Vedda population comes from coconut and wild game, both high in saturated fat.

The study of the Vedda population examined 207 adults between 20-83 years of age. A detailed medical history was taken of each subject, which included level of daily physical activity, dietary and smoking habits. A complete physical examination and blood analysis was performed with special attention to cardiovascular diseases. None of the subjects reported heart related problems despite the fact that 39% of the men smoked, and only 3.8% had elevated blood pressure. Electrocardiograms showed no evidence of heart disease.

Even with the high saturated fat diet, total cholesterol as well as triglyceride levels were comparable those of the Sri Lanka population. The chief difference is they consume little polyunsaturated fats and no vegetable oils.

In 1978, Sri Lanka had a very low rate of coronary heart disease as well, representing one (1) death per 100,000 of the population. As with most countries though, the importation of polyunsaturated vegetable oils increased over time and consequently, the use of coconut oil decreased as the result of a cheaper alternative to traditional coconut oil. According to WHO statistics from 2012, ischemic heart disease was (and still is) the leading cause of death in Sri Lanka, killing 32,6000 people per year. Today, Sri Lanka has a death rate from ischemic heart disease of 66 deaths per 100,000 which is in line with the countries in the lower end of the cardiovascular disease rate in figure 13. This is lower than the western countries, but still, this represents a 66% increase from 1978!

There are other populations with little cardiovascular disease and no vegetable oil consumption, despite their relatively high saturated fat diet. The Pukapuka and Tokalau populations live on atolls in the northern Cook Island. These Polynesians eat a diet that consists mainly of breadfruit, fish and coconuts, although pork and chicken are consumed occasionally. Flour, sugar and canned meats arrive by boat every couple of months. The diet is low on unsaturated fats and no vegetable oils.

The consumption of coconut is higher in the Tokalau (63%) than the Pukapuka (36%). Therefore, the amount of saturated fat is higher in the Tokalau, and is reflected by an increase of 35-40mg/dl of total cholesterol over the Pukapuka.

Biopsies from adipose tissue show both groups have 10-12% lauric acid (12:0 saturated fat), and 16-17% myristic acid (14:0 saturated fat). Total groups have tissue saturated fats of 52-53% while unsaturated fats constitute 47-48% of adipose fat. The unsaturated fats are mostly monounsaturated fats. This is compared to adipose tissue samples in New Zealand Europeans containing 34% saturated fat and 64% unsaturated fats.

Despite the high saturated fat diet, coronary heart disease is essentially non-existent. And there is no evidence that the high saturated fat diet has a harmful effect on either population, but strongly suggests the absence of vegetable oils in the diet may be responsible for the low incidence of cardiovascular disease.

In summary, we know that vegetable oils are deteriorated by repeated heating that leads to lipid peroxidation. The prolonged consumption of the repeatedly heated oil will increase blood pressure and total cholesterol. The omega-6 polyunsaturated fats and their metabolites cause vascular inflammation, as well as vascular changes, which predispose oneself to atherosclerosis. This vascular inflammation may be the triggering episode, leading to the cascading events that result in atherosclerosis. Continued consumption of omega-6 polyunsaturated fats and their metabolites leads to oxy-LDL formation and modification of the Apo B protein. This causes a recognition by tissue monocytes which engulf the LDL-particle and become trapped, leading ultimately to the deposits of cholesterol in the intima of the coronary arteries (and elsewhere). And this is repeated with every meal where polyunsaturated (and monounsaturated) fats are consumed, again due to the reactivity of the double bonds in unsaturated fats.

6. Lipid Peroxidation

Have you ever noticed the brown varnish-like gunk that form on the side of your pan after frying? Ever wonder what was in it and what it was doing to you once consumed? This is the result of heating unstable polyunsaturated oil undergoing a process of "polymerization". Polymerization is the chemical process where the individual fatty acids link together to form long chains. The linoleic fatty acid in polyunsaturated oils starts the chain reaction which continues forming the gunk that condenses on the side of pans, grill, etc. Linoleic fatty acid comprises 30 percent of peanut oil, 52 percent of soybean oil, and 60 percent of corn oil, and it degrades into other oxidation products such as free radicals, degraded fats, and oxidation products. According to one analysis, a total of 130 volatile compounds were isolated from a piece of fried chicken alone!

While it is beyond the scope of this book to analyze all potentially toxic end products resulting from heating polyunsaturated oils and their exposure to oxygen, we will analyze the major breakdown products and explore the health implications which are many.

Lipid peroxidation is involved in various and numerous pathological states including inflammation, atherosclerosis, neurodegenerative diseases, and cancer.

To understand the impact of polyunsaturated fats on the function of cellular structures, we must first look at the structure of fats. The term fat is used frequently both in every day conversation as well in scientific publications. In both cases, the term encompasses a large class of molecules with differing structures and functions. Unfortunately, results of numerous trials frequently do not take into account the complexity of the individual fat molecule, the three-dimensional structure, nor the degree conversion the molecule has undergone.

Saturated fatty acids are lipid molecules whose carbon atoms are saturated with hydrogen. Most saturated fatty acids are straight hydrocarbon chains with an even number of carbon atoms. The most common fatty acids contain 12–22 carbon atoms. Saturated fats are commonly found in animals, and are solid at room temperature. Lard, suet, tallow, and butter are common saturated animal fats; coconut and palm oil are two saturated vegetable oils. Saturated fats are generally more stable than the unsaturated fats due to the lack of the double bond.

Monounsaturated and Polyunsaturated fatty acids

Monounsaturated fatty acids have one carbon–carbon double bond. Oleic acid, present in olive oil, is a monounsaturated fat. When more than one area of the carbon chain can accept additional hydrogen atoms, the fat is said to be polyunsaturated.

Linoleic acid, an essential fatty acid found in safflower oil, soybean oil, and other vegetable oils, is an example of a polyunsaturated fat. Other oils of this category include peanut, corn, and cottonseed oils.

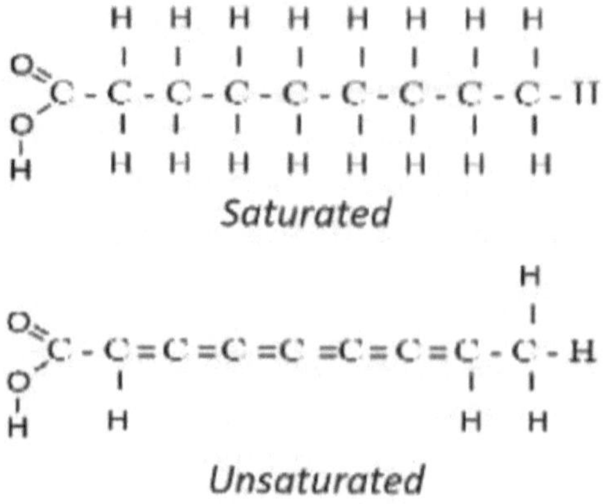

Saturated

Unsaturated

Figure 14: Saturated fatty acid vs. Polyunsaturated fatty acid. Polyunsaturated fats are characterized by the multiple double bonds.

This difference in double bonds is extremely important in understanding the differences in saturated and unsaturated fats and their effect on human metabolism. Unsaturated fats are unstable at room temperature and sensitive to interaction with oxygen, light, and heat. Less saturated vegetable oil oxidizes more than saturated oil. With the increase of unsaturation there is increase in primary oxidation products. These oxidation products incorporate into various aspects of the cell and are extremely toxic.

<u>Reactive Oxygen Species</u> (ROS) is a phrase used to describe a number of reactive molecules and free radicals derived from oxygen. These molecules, produced as byproducts during the mitochondrial electron transport of aerobic respiration, can cause havoc in the cell.

In general, harmful effects of reactive oxygen species on the cell are most often:

- damage of DNA
- oxidations of polyunsaturated fatty acids in lipids (lipid peroxidation)
- oxidations of amino acids in proteins
- oxidative deactivation of specific enzymes.

In particular, there are two prevalent ROS that profoundly affect lipids; hydroxyl radical (HO·) and hydroperoxyl (HO·2). The hydroxyl radical (HO·) is chemically most reactive species of activated oxygen. Enzymes in the cell, specifically catalase and superoxide dismutase (SOD) moderates the damaging effects by converting these compounds into oxygen and water. Most of the superoxide is converted to hydrogen peroxide by superoxide dismutase. However, this conversion is not always efficient, and residual peroxides persist in the cell. A cell produces around 50 hydroxyl radicals every second. In a full day, each cell would generate 4 million hydroxyl radicals, which are either neutralized, or live on to attack biomolecules. While ROS are produced as a product of normal cellular functioning, excessive amounts, can overwhelm the cellular defenses, and cause deleterious effects.

Lipid peroxidation is a degradation process involving the double bond(s) found in both mono and polyunsaturated fatty acids, causing a deterioration of food quality (odor, flavor, color, texture, toxicity). This is collectively known as turning "rancid". The well-known targets of damaging and potentially lethal peroxidative modification and glycolipids, phospholipids (PLs), and cholesterol (Ch).

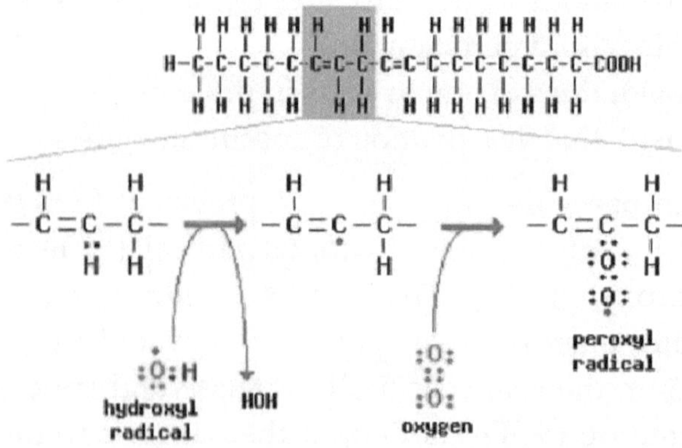

Figure 15: Lipid peroxidation reaction. A common target for peroxidation is the unsaturated fats in cellular membranes.

The overall process of lipid peroxidation consists of multiple steps where hydroxyl radical interacts with the polyunsaturated fatty acid (figure 15). Once lipid peroxidation is started, a chain reaction continues until termination products are produced.

Lipid peroxidation of unsaturated fatty acids produces a wide variety of oxidation products. The main primary products of lipid peroxidation are lipid hydroperoxides (LOOH). Among the many different aldehydes which can be formed as secondary products during lipid peroxidation, malondialdehyde (MDA), propanal, hexanal, and 4-hydroxynonenal (4-HNE) have been extensively studied. MDA appears to be the most mutagenic product of lipid peroxidation, whereas 4-HNE is the most toxic.

Lipid peroxidation is not limited to the cellular environment. During the frying process, cooking oil is exposed to an extremely high temperature in the presence of air and moisture. Under such conditions, a complex series of chemical reactions takes place. Repeatedly heating the cooking oils initiates a series of chemical reactions, modifying the fat constituents of cooking oil through oxidation, hydrolysis, polymerization, and isomerization, eventually resulting in lipid peroxidation. Lipid peroxidation generates a wide spectrum of volatile or non-volatile components, including free fatty acids, alcohols, aldehydes, ketones, hydrocarbons, *trans* isomers, cyclic and epoxy compounds. These toxic products are absorbed by the food, and eventually into the gastrointestinal tract and thereafter enter the systemic circulation.

<u>Malondialdehyde</u> (MDA) is a highly reactive three carbon di-aldehyde produced as a byproduct of polyunsaturated fatty acid peroxidation and arachidonic acid metabolism. MDA readily combines with several functional groups on molecules including proteins, lipoproteins, and DNA. Malondialdehyde is a

biomarker of lipid peroxidation that has been widely associated with food rancidity as well as many human diseases. It has been shown that interaction of low-density lipoprotein (LDL) with malondialdehyde abolishes the ability of the LDL receptor to recognize the modified lipoprotein.

There is an inverse relation between the severity of heart disease and MDA levels, supporting the hypothesis that free radical production is indeed involved in heart failure and is linked to its severity. Radovanovic *et al.*, noted that high plasma MDA concentration was a significant predictor of mortality in a study involving 120 patients with chronic heart failure. The patients with MDA above the cut-off had eight times higher mortality risk.

The predictive value of MDA for a cardiovascular event is also shown in the 634 patients from the *Prospective Randomized Evaluation of the Vascular Effects of Norvasc Trial*. Patients with MDA concentration in the highest levels were 3.3 time most likely to have a major vascular event (myocardial infarction—fatal, nonfatal, stroke), 4.1 times more likely for nonfatal vascular events (unstable angina), and 3.8 time for major vascular procedures (percutaneous interventions, coronary artery bypass grafting) as compared to the lowest levels.

4-Hydroxynonenal (4-HNE), is the major end product generated by decomposition of arachidonic acid and larger polyunsaturated fatty acids, through enzymatic or non-enzymatic processes. Phospholipids containing linoleic acid (LA, 18:2, *n*-6) and arachidonic acid (AA, 20:4, *n*-6) on cytoplasmic membranes or *n*-6 polyunsaturated fatty acids which are abundant in vegetable oils are considered the major source for 4-HNE production. 4-HNE is an extraordinarily reactive compound. 4-HNE is the most intensively studied lipid peroxidation end-product, in relation to its cytotoxic role inhibiting gene expression and promoting the development and progression of different diseases.

It has been established that High Density Lipoprotein (HDL) helps to protect against cardiovascular disease. As was discussed, HDL's physiologic role is the reverse cholesterol transport pathway, where HDL facilitates the removal of cholesterol from peripheral macrophages for delivery to the liver for excretion. In macrophages, HDL also protects against the generation of ROS, and promotes the production of anti-inflammatory cytokines. While increased levels of high-density lipoprotein (HDL)-cholesterol correlate with protection against cardiovascular disease, recent findings demonstrate that HDL function, rather than HDL-cholesterol levels, may be a better indicator of cardiovascular risk. Macrophages play a major role in the development and progression of atherosclerosis. It has been shown that modification of HDL with reactive aldehydes such as acrolein or 4-hydroxynonenal impairs macrophage migration, while modification of HDL with malondialdehyde promotes the generation of reactive oxygen species within macrophages. Impairing macrophage migration (or trapping) is a critical step in the progression of atherosclerosis.

9-hydroxy-10,12-octadecadienoic acid (9-HODE). The most prevalent fatty acid contained in LDL cholesterol is linoleic acid. When the LDL is oxidized, the linoleic acids in the lipoprotein are converted to hydroperoxides, which in turn are converted to 9-HODE. 9-HODE is extremely prevalent in oxidized LDL and is a good indicator of lipid peroxidation. In fact, 9-HODE is 20 times higher in young patients with atherosclerosis compared with healthy volunteers, and 30-fold to 100-fold greater in patients with atherosclerosis aged 69 to 94 compared with young healthy individuals.

Other compounds that are created in vegetable oils during processing are monochlorpropane-diols and glycidol esters (MCPDs). 3-monochloropropane-1,2-diol (3-MCPD) is a contaminant which occurs through food processing. It is formed in foods containing fat and salt when they are exposed to high temperatures during production. The formation of 3-MCPD in food is influenced by many factors, including temperature, pH, moisture content, sugar and lipid content. It is registered at the federal level as a _rodenticide_ with restricted use, under the name α-chlorohydrin!

Oxylipins are bioactive lipids generated by the oxidation of polyunsaturated fatty acids and are found throughout the body in all tissues, urine, and blood. So far, over 100 oxylipins have been identified and have overlapping roles. Oxylipins have been implicated in many cardiovascular disease pathologies, including: hyperlipidemia, hypertension, thrombosis, hemostasis,

Oxylipin	Physiological Effect
	Linoleic Acid derived
9-HODE	Present in oxidized LDL. Induces Macrophages
13-HODE	Prevents platelets from adhering to vascular endothelial cells.
9,10-DiHOME	Oxidative stress and endothelial inflammation
	Arachidonic Acid derived
PGD_2	Inhibits platelet aggregation
PGE_2	Implicated in cardiac ischemia and hypertrophy
PGF_{2a}	Induces vasoconstriction in coronary arteries. Is associated with cardiac hypertrophy
TXA_2	Induces vasoconstriction and platelet aggregation
TXB_2	High blood pressure and multiple cardiovascular effects
LTs	Atherosclerosis, endothelial dysfunction, intimal hyperplasia
5,6diHETrE	Associated with high blood pressure
11,12diHETrE	Associated with multiple cardiovascular events

Figure 16: Some of the Known Oxylipins and their cardiovascular effects.

and diabetes. Oxylipins, and more specifically the eicosanoids produced from arachidonic acid, have long been implicated in atherosclerosis, platelet aggregation, vascular constriction, and cardiac injury and dys function.

Although the oxylipins derived from arachidonic acid are the best characterized, oxylipins derived from other polyunsaturated fatty acids have also been implicated in cardiovascular disease. For example, oxylipins derived from linoleic acid have been associated with atherosclerosis and inflammation.

In a recent investigation of nearly 100 patients with cardiovascular disease, the prevalence of transient ischemic attacks, strokes, angina, and acute coronary syndrome was studied to determine whether plasma oxylipins were related to cardiovascular/ cerebrovascular events. They found that eight of the nearly 40 plasma oxylipins identified known to regulate vascular tone were significantly associated with these clinical events. For example, plasma 16-HETE was more than four times higher in patients that suffered from a cerebrovascular accident versus those that did not. Plasma 8,9-DiHETrE increased the odds by 92-fold of acute coronary syndrome.

7. Calcification

Vascular calcification was first recognized in the 19th century by Rudolph Virchow believing it was an extension to the bone making process. It wasn't until 100 years later that the group of Tanimura *et al.*, described the process of calcification of the intimal layer. Calcification of the coronary arteries has been correlated with atherosclerosis dating back to the 1940's. Indeed, cardiologists at that time utilized large red googles to maintain dark adaption so as to enable them to view calcium deposits on fluoroscopy screens. Today, arterial calcium can be measured with high-speed multi-slice computed tomography (CT) scans, which allows for measurement of both the density and extent

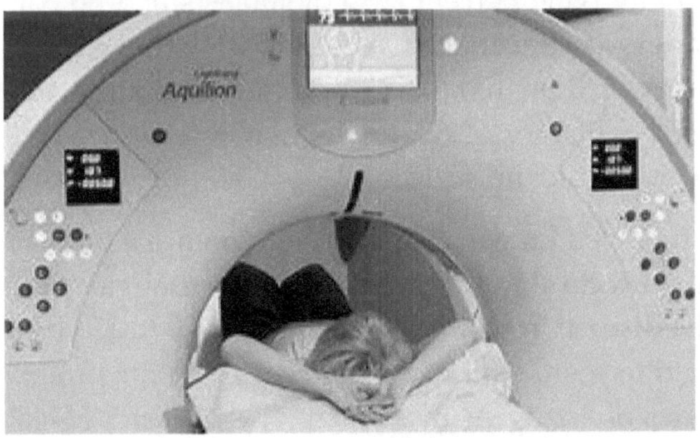

Figure 17: High-speed multi-slice computed tomography (CT).

of coronary calcification.

Most people 60 years and older have enlarging deposits of calcium mineral in their major arteries. The resulting calcification causes a reduction in both the size and elasticity of arteries thereby leading to high blood pressure, artery blockage, heart enlargement (hypertrophy), congestive heart failure, as well as my-ocardial ischemia (lack of blood supply). The extent of calcification is directly correlated to the amount of ath-erosclerotic plaque and is a predictor of cardiac disease and death.

The Pittsburgh, Pennsylvania, field center of the Cardiovascular Health studied 614 older adults aver-age age 80 years (range, 67 to 99 years), to determine the extent of their vascular calcification. They found calcium scores ranged from 0 to 5459, with an average score of 622 for men and 205 for women. Scores in-creased by age and were lower in blacks than in whites. Only Nine percent (9%) of subjects had no cor-onary artery calcification (CAC), and 31% (n=190) had a score lower than 100. It is important to note in this study that a history of cardiovascular disease was as-sociated with calcium score.

It is well known that whether you are a male or a female affects the development of arterial calcifica-tion. The disease in women is delayed by 10 to 15 years compared to men, which is probably due to the protec-tive effects of estrogens in women. The *Women's Health Initiative* looked at 1,064 females aged 50 to 59 years randomized to either estrogen therapy or placebo. The estrogen group had a significantly lower CAC score (average of 83.1) compared to placebo.

The CADRE (*Coeur Artères Drepanocytose*) study evaluated the degree of CAC in 108 human hearts taken from patients who died of sudden cardiac death. When the ages of the subjects we divided by decades, the degree of calcification was greater in men compared to women up to the 6th decade of life. By the 7th decade, the degree of calcification was similar. They also observed that the degree of calcification was 3 times greater in post, versus pre-menopausal women.

There is also a strong racial variation in amount of calcification. In the MESA (*Multi-Ethnic Study of Atherosclerosis*), a total of 6,814 whites, African Americans, Hispanic, and Chinese people aged 45 to 84 years, with no history of clinical cardiovascular disease, were studied for coronary calcification. The prevalence of coronary calcification (Agatston score >0) was 70.4% for white males, 52.1% for African-American males, 56.5% for Hispanic Males, and 59.2% for Chinese men. In females, the same pattern emerged. They observed that the extent of CAC was greater in Caucasians versus African Americans for every decade.

The Agatston score is the sum of all calcified lesions that takes into consideration total calcified area as well as maximum density of the calcification. Although other methods of scoring have been used, the Agatston score is the gold standard. The presence of minimal CAC (i.e., CAC score 1 to 10) increases the risk of experiencing a coronary heart disease (CHD) event by 3-

fold as compared with the absence of CAC.

Grading of coronary artery disease (based on total calcium score)

- no evidence of CAD: 0 calcium score
- minimal: 1-10
- mild: 11-100
- moderate: 101-400
- severe: >400

The depositing of calcium phosphate is the key feature of cardiovascular calcification, and can be seen in the blood vessels, myocardium (lining of the interior of the heart), as well as the heart valves. There is a plethora of articles showing vascular calcification is strongly correlated to atherosclerosis. There are various risk factors that contribute to the development of vascular calcification. Aging is the major risk factor for vascular calcification, while others include diabetes, chronic kidney disease, elevated cholesterol, high blood pressure, being male, white, and a smoker.

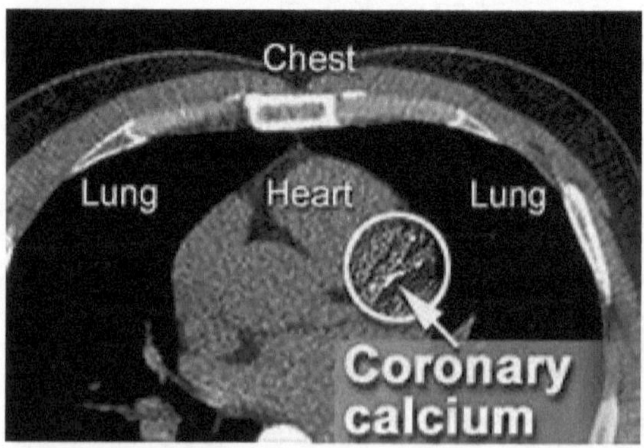

Figure 18: High-speed multi-slice computed tomography showing coronary calcification.

Arterial calcification is divided into intimal calcification, the predominant form of calcification in coronary artery plaques; and medial calcification, which mostly affects peripheral arteries and aortas. Intimal calcification usually develops with progression of atherosclerosis, and may cause coronary ischemic events. Medial calcification is independent of atherosclerosis, and predominantly develops along elastic fibers. Consequently, medial calcification promotes arterial stiffness, and increases systolic blood pressure, resulting in enlargement of the left ventricle of the heart leading to heart failure.

It is believed that the death of smooth muscle cells of the artery is the driving force for the early stage of calcification. Calcification begins within the core of dead cells within the atherosclerotic plaque. Oxidized lipoprotein cholesterol is particularly toxic to the macrophage, and, if present in sufficient quantity, can cause death of the cholesterol filled macrophage (foam cell). Immune cells accelerate the process by producing antibodies that recognize oxidized LDL. Smooth muscle cells then migrate into the intima, proliferate, and initiate the formation of a fibrous cap. The combination of oxidative stress, and cholesterol overload induce macrophage cell death. Interestingly, more than 40% of dead cells in an inflamed atherosclerotic lesion are macrophages.

Vesicles similar to the endothelial particles are released by dead or dying macrophages and smooth muscle cells. These vesicles provide the scaffolding for the start of calcification. This is followed by an infiltration of macrophages which also undergoes cell death and calcification creating the downward spiral of increasing calcification.

Not all cardiovascular medication reduces coronary calcification. Most surprisingly, statins are found to promote the progression of coronary calcification. This is unexpected given that statins are marketed for their cardiovascular protective effects, based on the premise that elevated cholesterol is associated with calcification. Similarly, high intensity exercise paradoxically accelerates coronary artery calcification, even though exercise is associated with a reduction in mortality in patients with coronary artery calcification. Highly intensive statin therapy has been shown to be associated with plaque volume reduction albeit by a small amount, with volume regression from baseline (0.6%), whereas both low or no-statin therapy were associated with percent plaque volume progression (0.8%).

In other studies, statins have also been shown to be a risk factor for calcium progression. The SATURN (*Study of Coronary Atheroma by Intravascular Ultrasound: Effect of Rosuvastatin Versus Atorvastatin*) trial showed an increase in dense calcium volume in 71 patients treated with high-dose rosuvastatin or atorvastatin for 24 months. A recent meta-analysis and systematic review of the impact of statin therapy on coronary plaque composition suggested a significant increase in dense calcium only in patients taking statins.

Vitamin K

Vascular calcification can be considered to be an imbalance between the mechanisms that promote and inhibit the deposition of calcium in the vascular wall. In this regard the vitamin K plays an important role as an inhibitor of soft tissue calcification. Vitamin K is a fat-soluble vitamin including vitamin K1 (phylloquinone) from green leafy vegetables and vitamin K2 (menaquinones) from dairy products, meat and egg yolk.

Vitamin K functions as a cofactor for an enzyme which converts glutamate into gammacarboxyglutamate (Gla). Gla-containing proteins are involved in, among other things, the coagulation of blood, inhibition of arterial calcification, and vascular smooth muscle cell death and movement, which is considered protective against vascular injury. The Gla Protein is involved in both medial as well as intimal calcification, and low vitamin K status has been associated with both types of calcifications.

Vitamin K-dependent proteins (VKDPs) are a group of proteins that require vitamin K to function. A total of 17 VKDPs have been identified in humans. Of these, there are three that function in cardiac artery calcification: Growth arrest-specific protein 6 (Gas 6), Gla-rich protein (GRP) and periostin. Gas 6 and GRP are both effective in protecting blood vessels from calcification, while MGP plays a beneficial role in vascular calcification and various pathological processes. Evidence suggests Gas 6 is significantly secreted by vascular smooth muscle cells in human atherosclerotic plaques, yet there is no secretion in healthy blood vessels. Therefore, Gas 6 acts as a protective factor in human atherosclerosis.

The inhibition of vitamin-K by vitamin K blockers (such as warfarin) results in extensive arterial calcification in experimental animals. In mice, warfarin accelerates both medial and intimal calcification of atherosclerotic plaque. Observational studies show that long-term use of vitamin-K blockers is associated with increased coronary calcifications.

Vitamin K supplementation presents an attractive treatment option to reduce vascular calcifications. In rats, dietary supplementation with high doses of either phylloquinone (vitamin K1) or menaquinone-4 (vitamin K2) resulted in the regression of arterial calcifications indued by warfarin. In mice, a low-dose of vitamin K-2 along with warfarin reduced the development of calcification.

Observational studies in humans have shown an improvement in CAC with vitamin K-2 in healthy elderly. Taking vitamin K-1 supplements alone was shown to slow the progression of CAC, and had a beneficial effect on vascular stiffness in healthy adults with coronary artery calcification after 3 years of follow-up. Those patients assigned to vitamin K1 had a 6% less progression in CAC than those in the control group.

Dalmeijer *et al.* performed a randomized, double blind, placebo-controlled trial to investigate the effect of menaquinone-7 (MK-7) supplementation and found that MK-7 improves arterial stiffness and elastic properties of the carotid artery. In another study, Teresa R Haugsgjerd, *et al* (2020) followed participants in the community-based *Hordaland Health Study* from 1997 - 1999 through 2009 to evaluate associations between intake of vitamin K and the incident of (new onset) CHD. Those participants with a higher intake of vitamin K-2 had a lower risk of CHD, while there was no association between intake of vitamin K1 and CHD.

<u>Vitamin D</u>

Vitamin D is found in nature in two forms: D2 (ergocalciferol) and D3 (cholecalciferol). Vitamin D3, also known as "the sunshine vitamin," is either synthetized in the skin from sun light, or consumed in the form of oily fish or in the form of vitamin supplements. Vitamin D2 is found in plants. The vitamin is converted in the liver and kidney to calcitriol, and acts on specific tissues through vitamin D receptors found in the intestines, bones, and kidneys. Vitamin D functions to increase calcium absorption from the intestines, and to promote calcium deposits in bone. However, vitamin D receptors are also found in other tissues, including vascular smooth muscle cells, and endothelial cells. Vitamin D receptors decreases with age.

Low levels of vitamin D2 are associated with endothelial dysfunction, inflammation, increased vascular stiffness as well as high coronary artery calcium scores. In addition, vitamin D2 deficiency affects vascular functions by aggravating atherosclerosis, while treatment with vitamin D2 may have protective effects on atherosclerosis. Low vitamin D2 levels have been found to be associated with early signs of atherosclerosis such as increased carotid intima-media wall thickness.

Clinical studies also suggest a possible relationship between vitamin D2 deficiency and vascular calcification. Satilmis *et al* (2015) looked at 98 patients with coronary atherosclerosis and compared finding with 110, age and gender matched subjects with normal findings. Patients with subclinical atherosclerosis had significantly higher serum total cholesterol, triglycerides, C. Reactive Protein, and lower serum vitamin D2 levels in comparison with controls.

Only a few clinical studies have studied the benefits of vitamin D in the treatment of cardiovascular disease. In one study, the results indicated a significant reduction in CAD and vascular inflammation. However, two large scale studies failed to demonstrate a beneficial effect of vitamin D on cardiovascular disease. These two studies by Seibert *et al.* and Sokol *et al.* had a study period of 12 weeks and did not show significant changes in endothelial markers, blood pressure, inflammation or blood cholesterol. Since atherosclerosis occurs over a lifetime, perhaps a longer duration of intervention is necessary.

In a small study by Arnson *et al.*, five days of Vitamin D3 treatment attenuated some inflammatory and endothelial markers. Similarly, Raygan *et al.* found reduced vascular inflammation and metabolic improvements in diabetic patients supplemented with 12 weeks of vitamin D. A comprehensive 2019 meta-analysis by Barbarawi *et al.* including 83,000 participants did not find beneficial cardiovascular outcomes following vitamin D supplementation. Clearly, additional clinical trials are necessary of sufficient duration and dosage to determine whether Vitamin D has any benefit in cardiovascular disease.

8 Dysbiosis

Humans have evolved alongside the vast numbers of microorganisms that inhabit the body and the gut. In fact, the average human being has as many bacterial cells as his/her own cell numbers! These organisms are mostly populated in the colon, harboring over 100,000,000,000(10^{10}-10^{12}) colony-forming units per gram of feces. It turns out that humans carry between 500-1,000 different bacterial species with the majority belonging in only two distinct phyla: *Firmicutes* and *Bacteroidetes*. Other phyla present to a lesser extent include: *Actinobacteria, Proteobacteria, Fusobacteria, Spirochaete and Verrucomicrobia* (figure19). Only a restricted set of bacterial populations in nature have been identified in the human body, while approximately 80% of the human bacteria identified by genomic sequencing, are considered uncultivable in the laboratory. Although some prevalent bacterial species in normal individuals are now identified by using whole genome sequencing, more than 60% of species remain unknown

This complex community of bacteria serves a variety of functions from food digestion, to energy supply, to immune response. While the largest populations are relatively constant between individuals, there is diversity with each individual sheltering over a

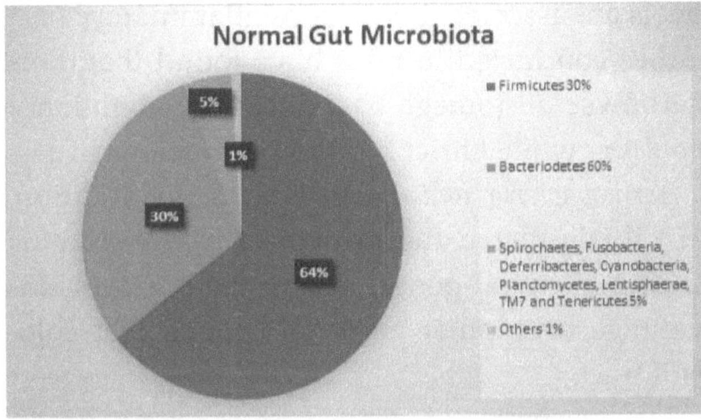

Figure 19: The gut normally has a divided population of 60% Bacteriodetes, 30% Firmicutes, and 6% other species. Dysbiosis refers to any imbalance within the gut flora

hundred distinctive species.

Given the symbiotic relationship between these bacteria and intestinal well-being, it should come as little surprise that factors affecting the gut microbiota, or gut flora, would in turn affect the host. A functioning microbiota is crucial to maintaining a balance of local and systemic homeostasis. A disturbance in the population of microbiota results in gut <u>dysbiosis</u>.

Dysbiosis refers to any imbalance within the gut flora. Numerous studies have shown that an imbalance in dietary PUFAs can lead to dysbiosis. And as you would expect, an individual's omega-6 to omega-3 ratio seen in their adipose tissue profile is reflected in changes in the microbiota. Studies have shown that animals with high tissue n-3 PUFA levels are associated with anti-inflammatory gut bacteria, while high n-6 PUFA levels are associated with pro-inflammatory bacteria. Studies conducted in mice have found that diets rich in safflower oil (omega-6) reduces the abundance of *Bacteroidetes*, while enriching the populations of *Firmicutes, Actinobacteria and Proteobacteria*. In addition, safflower oil stimulated the growth of δ-*Proteobacteria* by enhancing bacterial genes, giving them a competitive advantage over other bacterial groups that colonize the GI tract.

Mice fed a diet rich in omega-6 PUFAs (corn oil) results in bacterial overgrowth and dysbiosis. The high n-6 PUFA diet, is associated with bacterial invasion of the intestinal epithelial cell layer. Corn oil supplementation caused hyperinsulinemia.

Inflammation is the result of the secretion of lipopolysaccharide (LPS) from gram negative bacteria. LPS is the major component of the outer membrane of the bacteria, and when released, is considered an endotoxin due to its potent stimulatory effect on the immune system. The pro-inflammatory bacteria, commonly found in animals consuming a high omega-6 diet, produce greater amounts of LPS while the bacterium of high omega-3 fed animals do not produce nearly as much LPS, and thus have less inflammatory significance.

Atherosclerosis

There is significant evidence that the gut microbiota is involved in the development of atherosclerosis, and to support this claim are numerous studies that implicate microbial byproducts in atherogenesis. Specific bacterial DNA has been identified in atherosclerotic plaques which are linked to bacteria found in oral or gut samples from patients with atherosclerosis. DNA sequencing of fecal samples has found the *Bacteroides* were diminished and *Ruminococcus* overgrown in atherosclerotic patients.

Lipopolysaccharides, as discussed earlier, are released from gram-negative bacteria which then leads to a chronic inflammatory state that accelerates atherosclerosis in humans and rodents. For example, delivery of C. *pneumoniae* to the vessel wall of carotid arteries in mice increases the development of atherosclerosis. Repeated intravenous and intraperitoneal administration of LPS accelerates atherosclerosis in rabbits and mice.

Specifically, bacterial components such as lipopolysaccharides can promote the formation of foam cells, which are a major component of atherosclerotic plaque. As discussed earlier, foam cells are macrophages that have engulfed excessive amounts of modified low-density lipoprotein (LDL) cholesterol in an attempt to remove it from the bloodstream. The LDL then undergoes oxidation through enzymatic attack or reaction with reactive oxygen species to produce ox-

LDLs. The accumulation of ox-LDLs within the arterial wall stimulates endothelial cells to express cell adhesion molecules (such as vascular cell adhesion molecule-1) and chemokines (such as monocyte chemoattractant protein-1), that cause monocytes to adhere to the endothelium.

As we discussed previously, the human body has processes to defend against excess cholesterol buildup in tissues such as reverse cholesterol transport (RCT). RCT is a process by which excess cholesterol is brought to the liver to be converted into bile acids (BAs). The transport of cholesterol is mediated by apolipoprotein A1 on high density lipoproteins (HDLs) which bind to cholesterol to transport to the liver. Gut dysbiosis can overwhelm the reverse transport mechanisms and therefore promote the formation of foam cells, specifically by inducing metabolic endotoxemia. Metabolic endotoxemia is a condition characterized by an increased presence of LPS in circulation.

Omega-6 induced dysbiosis is associated with reduced presence of *bifidobacteria*, which normally promotes the intestinal barrier. Dysbiosis also results in the reduced expression of intestinal tight junction proteins, further increasing intestinal permeability. This allows for increased levels of LPS to enter circulation, which goes on to promote inflammation and foam cell formation.

In addition to the metabolism-independent pathway, dysbiosis can exert pro-atherosclerotic effects by altering the generation of a number of metabolites.

Specifically, dysbiosis has been shown to affect the metabolism of bile acids, as well as the production of trimethylamine-n-oxide (TMAO), and butyrate.

Bile Acids are produced from cholesterol and aid in the digestion of dietary fats. Formation of bile acids is the major pathway for the breakdown of cholesterol. Bile acids have two important functions in atherosclerosis: they are the major path for cholesterol elimination, and bile acids exhibit significant protective effect against atherosclerosis effects.

The gut microbiota regulates the bile acid pathway through their bacterial bile-salt hydrolase (BSH) activity, which is required in the formation of secondary bile acids. The primary bile acids are synthesized from cholesterol in the liver, and are released into the small intestine. Gut microbiota metabolizes the primary bile acids to form secondary bile acids. Bile acid transporters reabsorb 95% of bile acids from the intestine, which are then recycled by the liver. But, since secondary BAs are less soluble, they are less likely to be reabsorbed. Therefore, they are more likely to be excreted, providing a pathway for cholesterol elimination. This cycle is called the enterohepatic circulation of bile acids (figure 20).

In dysbiosis, there is a decline in bacterial bile-salt hydrolase activity which leads to less primary bile acid conversion and consequently more bile acids reabsorbed. Due to its role in regulating BA signaling, reduced bacterial BSH activity can lead to the accumulation of cholesterol, promoting the formation of foam cells, and ultimately, atherosclerotic plaque.

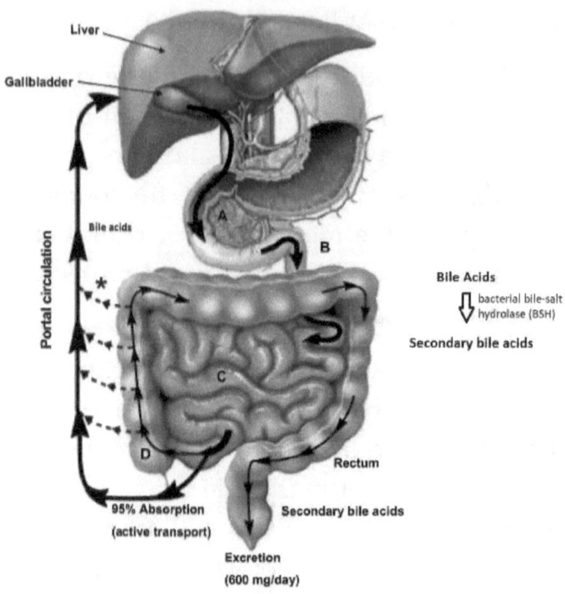

Figure 20: The enterohepatic circulation of bile acids. The primary bile acids are synthesized from cholesterol in the liver, and are released into the small intestine. Gut microbiota metabolize the primary bile acids to form secondary bile acids. Bile acid transporters reabsorb 95% of bile acids from the intestine, which are then recycled by the liver.

p-cresyl sulfate, is another bacterial metabolite which has been shown to readily penetrate the endothelial cell membrane and cause endothelial damage. p-cresyl sulfate induces the shedding of the endothelial microparticles we discussed earlier. Elevated plasma levels of p-cresyl sulfate are associated with the high concentrations of endothelial microparticles. These microparticles are related to increased arterial stiffness and act as pro-thrombotic and pro-inflammatory mediators.

The role of *p*-cresyl sulfate in mediating the release of the endothelial microparticles was confirmed by *in vitro* studies using cultured human endothelial cells. There is a correlation with elevated *p*-cresyl sulfate in plasma and the risk of cardiovascular disease. It is believed that *p*-cresyl may accumulate in vascular endothelial and smooth muscle cells, and induce oxidative stress through the production of radical oxygen species (ROS), thereby resulting in the development of cytotoxicity.

The other widely studied toxin generated by the gut microbiota is indoxyl sulfate. Indoxyl sulfate is a byproduct of the intestinal microbial flora and has been shown to promote the progression of renal and cardiovascular disease by inducing oxidative stress, inflammation and fibrosis.

In addition to atherosclerosis, dysbiosis can contribute to the progression of hypertension or high blood pressure. As an artery constricts, the inner diameter of the vessel decreases, thereby increasing peripheral vascular resistance resulting in elevated blood pressure. Gut dysbiosis contributes to hypertension through ox-LDL-induced vasoconstriction. Studies have demonstrated that patients with chronic heart failure and coronary artery diseases have decreased levels of vasodilators and increased vasoconstrictors. Ox-LDL affects the balance between vasoconstrictors and vasodilators through modulation of nitric oxide (NO). Ox-LDL is associated with the inhibition and decreased activity of NO synthase, the enzyme responsible for the conversion of L-arginine to form NO. With decreased production of NO there is less vasodilation leading to elevated blood pressure. In addition, ox-LDL can stimulate an increased production of endothelin-1 which has a vasoconstrictive effect. The higher levels of endothelin-1 the higher the amount of vasoconstriction, again leading to hypertension.

Another major site for microbiota colonization is the mouth. The microorganisms found in the oral cavity constitute the second-largest bacterial community after the gut. A high abundance of pathogenic bacteria in the oral cavity can lead to inflammatory diseases, such as periodontal disease, which has been linked to systemic inflammation and to atherosclerosis. The link between periodontitis and cardiovascular disease development was demonstrated in numerous studies, and treatment of periodontitis has been shown to substantially decrease the level of pro-inflammatory C-Reactive protein in patients with atherosclerosis. The oral pathogen Porphyromonas gingivalis increases atherosclerosis in mice compared to uninfected controls. Interestingly, when mice were immunized with killed *Porphyromonas gingivalis*, the accumulation of immune cells in atherosclerotic plaques was prevented.

Maintaining a Healthy Microbiota

The correction of dysbiosis is a promising area of cardiovascular research. It is intriguing that atherosclerosis may be treated through a reversal of dysbiosis. And diet is a major factor which shapes the gut microbiota. A simple means of reversing gut dysbiosis is through the reduction of the omega-6/omega-3 ratio in the diet. Elimination of omega-6 PUFAs from the diet will eliminate pro-inflammatory bacteria from the gut. Omega-3 PUFAs (EPA and DHA) can reversed bacterial overgrowth and reduced inflammation by recruiting regulatory T-cells to the small intestine. However, there is not a similar protection by saturated fatty acids.

Mice fed a diet high in omega-6 fatty acids exhibit higher levels of endotoxins in the blood, and systemic low-grade inflammation, while omega-3 fatty acids dramatically reduced the endotoxin load and inflammatory symptoms. Ghosh *et al.*, (2013) observed that feeding high-fat diets rich in n-6 PUFA promoted bacterial overgrowth, but depleted microbes from the *Bacteroidetes* and *Firmicutes* phyla. This change in the microbiota corresponded with increased body mass, with infiltration of macrophages and neutrophils. Fish oil supplementation restored the microbiota, reduced the inflammatory cell infiltration, and promoted regulatory T-cell recruitment. However, fish oil supplementation was associated with increased oxidative stress, evident by the increased presence of 4-hydroxynonenal, a product of lipid peroxidation. Interestingly, these effects are eliminated by antibiotic therapy thereby suggesting direct involvement by the gut microbiota. Elevated tissue omega-3 fatty acids enhance secretion of intestinal alkaline phosphatase (IAP), which induces changes in the gut bacteria population resulting in decreased lipopolysaccharide production.

Prebiotics are specialized plant fibers that selectively stimulate the growth of healthy bacteria in the gut. They are found mostly in fruits and vegetables, especially those that contain complex carbohydrates, such as fiber and resistant starch. Plant polyphenols travel through the gut without being modified, and have been able to influence the gut microbiota composition. Zhen-Lin Liao and colleagues (2016) treated atherosclerotic mice with tea polyphenols. They observed the total cholesterol and low-density lipoprotein cholesterol (LDL-C) were decreased significantly after tea polyphenol administration. In addition, the tea polyphenol diet also decreased the plaque area in the atherosclerotic lesions. The use of polyphenols will be further discussed in chapter 10.

Probiotics are live microorganisms that, when administered in adequate amounts can correct dysbiosis. The most common probiotic products are lactobacilli and bifidobacterial strains. Probiotics present an interesting means for treating elevated serum cholesterol levels. Current research on probiotics has been heavily focused on *lactobacilli* strains. There have been several clinical studies showing the beneficial effects of probiotics, including *Lactobacillus plantarum*, *Lactobacillus rhamnosus*, and *Lactobacillus curvatus* in terms of reducing the risk of development of coronary artery disease. Naruszewicz *et al.* (2002) administered *L. plantarum* (50 million CFU) to thirty-six healthy volunteers for six weeks and concluded that *L. plantarum* administration leads to a reduction in cardiovascular disease risk factors. Specifically, they noted a significant decrease in blood pressure and significantly reduced adhesion of monocytes in human endothelial cells.

A meta-analysis by Mo *et al.* (2019) indicates that the use of probiotics significantly lowers total cholesterol and low-density lipoprotein (LDL) cholesterol in hypercholesterolemic adults. Niamah *et al.* (2017) also noted that soy milk fermented with *S. thermophilis, L. acidophilus* and *B. bifidum* decreased the blood levels of cholesterol and triglyceride compared with control. Malik *et al.* (2018) report that *L. plantarum* supplementation improved vascular endothelial function and reduces inflammatory biomarkers in men with stable

Intervention	Outcome
Administration of Lactobacillus rhamnosus GG in high fat-fed mice	Reduction in atherosclerotic plaque size and cholesterol levels
Administration of Lactobacillus rhamnosus GG in high-fat subjected obese mice	Normalization of dyslipidemia, decrease in triglycerides, cholesterol and reduction subcutaneous adipose tissues
Administration of Lactobacillus rhamnosus GR-1 in coronary artery occlusion model in rats	Attenuation of left ventricular hypertrophy, and improvement in systolic and diastolic left ventricular function
Administration of Lactobacillus plantarum in diet-induced hypercholesterolemia model in mice	Decrease in cholesterol levels
Administration of Lactobacillus plantarum 299v in CAD patients	Improvement in the vascular endothelial function
Administration of Bacteroides vulgatus and Bacteroides dorei in atherosclerosis-prone mice	Attenuation of the development of atherosclerosis
Maintenance of mice in germ-free conditions	More severe atherosclerosis
Use of clarithromycin in CAD patients	Increased risk of mortality and morbidity

Figure 21: Probiotics and outcomes. Probiotics have been demonstrated to reduce cholesterol levels, improve vascular endothelium function, and attenuate the development of atherosclerosis.

coronary artery disease.

There is an abundance of animal studies showing the benefits of probiotics in reversing dysbiosis and improving cardiovascular markers. In high-fat fed mice, administration of *Lactobacillus rhamnosus* was shown to both reduce atherosclerotic plaque as well as cholesterol levels. Another study also showed the efficacy of orally administrated *Lactobacillus rhamnosus* in decreasing in the levels of triglycerides as well as cholesterol in high-fat fed obese mice. Interestingly, the administration of *Lactobacillus rhamnosus* significantly lessened the development of left ventricular enlargement and improved heart function in a coronary artery occlusion model in rats. In mice fed at high fat diet, administration of *Lactobacillus rhamnosus* was shown to reduce atherosclerotic plaque as well as cholesterol levels.

Moreover, administration of *Lactobacillus rhamnosus* significantly lessened the development of left ventricular hypertrophy and improved function in coronary artery occlusion model in rats. The hypocholesterolemia effects of *Lactobacillus plantarum* have also been reported in diet-induced hypercholesterolemia model in mice.

This is but a small sample of the numerous studies that have been published in recent years showing the intense interest in the role of gut microorganisms in the pathophysiology of cardiovascular disease. Bacteria in the can either produce beneficial effects in cardiovascular disease either directly in the form of oral administration of probiotics, or indirectly by acting on fiber-rich food in the form of prebiotics to produce important cardioprotective aspects. The harmful effects of gut microbiota in cardiovascular disease are due to alteration in their composition with a significant decrease in *Bacteroidetes* and an increase in *Firmicutes, Escherichia, Shigella,* and *Enterococcus species*. The altered bacteria may produce potentially toxic metabolites, including trimethylamine-N-oxide (TMAO). Indeed, the fasting plasma levels of TMAO are directly correlated to increased risk of major cardiovascular events, and it is a potential biomarker to predict the onset of atherosclerosis, as will be discussed in the next chapter.

9   Trimethylamine N-oxide

While different bacterial metabolites have been linked to atherosclerosis, we will focus on one in this chapter that has garnered much attention: *trimethylamine-N-oxide* (TMAO). Many studies have shown a close association between TMAO and the development of cardiovascular as well as other diseases. Different populations of gut bacteria have varying abilities to generate TMAO. TMAO levels have been found to closely correlate with certain human gut microbial bacteria. For example, in gut dysbiosis, where more *trimethylamine* (TMA)-producing bacteria are prevalent, higher levels of TMAO are observed, and therefore an increase in CVD risk. Higher TMAO plasma concentrations have been found to be associated with the species *Prevotella*, as opposed to *Bacteroides*.

The gut microbiota is responsible for the generation of TMA, by metabolizing choline from the diet to TMA. TMA is absorbed in the intestines, then metabolized to TMAO by the enzyme flavin monooxygenase (FMO) in the liver. Thus, the gut microbiota is a critical step in the pathogenesis of TMAO-induced atherosclerosis. As evidence of the role of the microbiota in TMA production, it has been shown that antibiotics reduce TMAO synthesis by blocking the conversion of L-carnitine to TMA governed by the gut bacteria (figure 22).

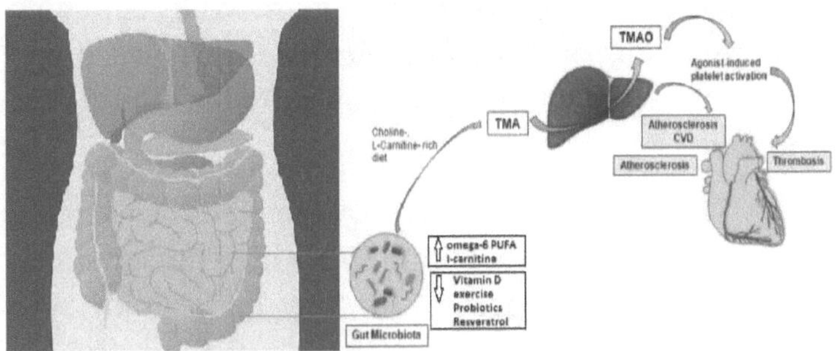

Figure 22: Production of TMA by gut microbiota. TMA is absorbed in the intestines and converted to TMAO in the liver.

However, because of side effects of antibiotics, the utility of this therapeutic approach is limited. Therefore, the identification of therapeutic interventions with either antimicrobial effects to inhibit gut microbiota, or reverse gut dysbiosis, would be useful for the prevention and treatment of TMAO induced atherosclerosis.

Only a small fraction of the bacteria in the gut (less than 1%) have the genes required for TMA production. However, even very low concentrations of these microorganisms seem to be sufficient for TMA production. The presence of increased TMA and TMAO levels has been associated with higher activity of bacterial members of the phylum *Firmicutes* and *Proteobacteria*, which are known producers of this metabolite. Moreover, TMA and TMAO levels have been linked to an elevated *Firmicutes/Bacteroidetes* ratio with higher levels of *Firmicutes* and lower levels of *Bacteroidetes* due to the inability of Bacteroidetes to produce TMA. A diet rich in safflower oil (omega-6) reduces the abundance of *Bacteroidetes*, while enriching the populations of *Firmicutes, Actinobacteria and Proteobacteria* again implicating polyunsaturated fats in the process of CVD.

The majority of TMAO in the blood is excreted unchanged in the urine within 24 hours. The remaining TMAO is changed back to TMA by the action of the enzyme TMAO reductase. Dietary choline and L-carnitine are the two principal precursors of TMAO. Choline, free choline and choline esters, such as phosphatidylcholine (lecithin), can be found in egg yolks, liver, meats, high-fat dairy products, as well as some certain nuts and beans. Choline is an essential nutrient for human, required for maintaining cell membranes and neurotransmission. L-carnitine another dietary precursor of TMAO, is found mostly in red meat and dairy products. L-carnitine is also an essential nutrient responsible for fatty acid transport.

Despite the prevalence of choline in the diet, a study investigating the TMAO production of 46 different foods found only fish (other sea-products) gave rise to significant increases in urinary trimethylamine and N-oxide. Ingestion of fruits, vegetables, cereal and dairy produce, and meats have no measurable effects. Yu *et al.* (2019) demonstrated that TMAO is strongly associated with deep-fried meat but not with red meat or poultry. In another study comparing meat and fish with the effect on TMAO production, fish was shown to induce a two-fold increase in urinary TMAO compared to meat. Five papers support the finding that ingestion of meats has no measurable effects on plasma or urinary TMAO. To put this into perspective, halibut generates over 107 times as much TMAO as red meat. It seems obvious that if any foods should be singled out for the production of TMAO, it should be seafoods. In many marine species, TMA acts as a protein stabilizer. The oxidized form decomposes into trimethylamine (TMA) which is responsible for the characteristic odor of putrefied fish. The free TMAO from seafood may be absorbed directly into the blood circulation without metabolism by the gut microbiome.

So why pick on red meat? A 1983 finding from Steven Zeisel *et.al.*, showed that high-dose choline and carnitine, but not lecithin, generated TMAO. Eight ounces of carnitine-rich foods, like red meat, produced no more TMAO than common fruits and vegetables. Seafoods, by contrast, led to large increases in TMAO. There is no clear evidence that beef produces more or less TMAO than any of the fruits and vegetables tested. Here (figure 23) we see that none of the meats tested were statistically different from vegetables, and that there is no relationship to the "redness" of the meat, with chicken having an almost identical value to beef. We see that bread, cheese and eggs all produced numerically (but not statistically) higher values than beef

Several lifestyle factors such as diet and exer-

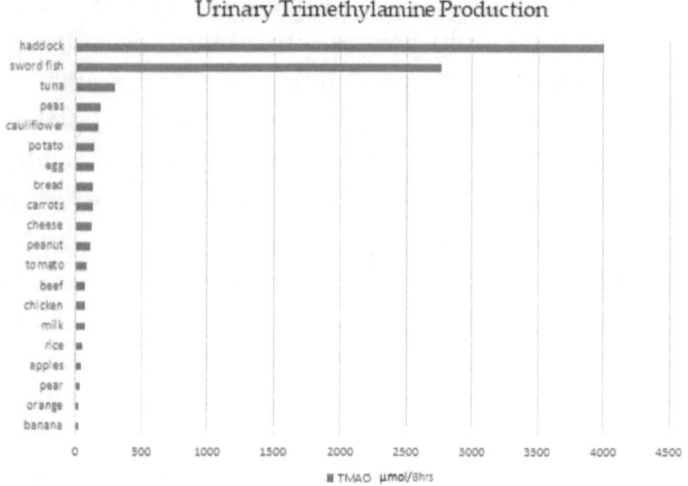

Figure 23: TMAO production in different foods.

cise may exert profound effects on the shift in gut microbial composition and gut microbiota-derived TMAO production. For example, Erickson *et al.*, (2019) found that a 12-week hypocaloric diet along with exercise decreased TMAO levels. Similar findings were observed by Leal-Witt *et al.*, (2018) in 34 obese children after a 6-month lifestyle intervention. Interestingly, the change in TMAO concentrations following intervention were not related to choline intake, but were correlated instead with fiber intake. Yet, Randrianarisoa *et al.*, (2016) found that TMAO levels did not change during the lifestyle intervention.

A significant effect of increased TMAO levels is the systemic accumulation of cholesterol by inhibiting hepatic bile acid synthesis. As you may recall from chapter 8, primary bile acids are synthesized from cholesterol in the liver and further metabolized by the gut microbiota into secondary bile acids in what is termed as the enterohepatic circulation of bile acids.

TMAO is also implicated in the process of atherosclerosis development by promoting macrophage migration, as well as transformation of macrophage into foam cell. TMAO augments the accumulation of ox-LDL, leading to more macrophage cells being transformed into foam cells. In addition, TMAO increases the expression of inflammatory cytokines. When responding to inflammatory activation, macrophages penetrate the endothelium and accumulate in vessel intima, contributing to the atherosclerotic plaque formation.

In 2013, Tang *et al.* published an article in the New England Journal of Medicine demonstrating the critical role of dietary choline and gut microbiota in TMAO production. The authors measured plasma and urinary levels of TMAO and plasma choline in healthy participants before and after the suppression of intestinal microbiota with oral broad-spectrum antibiotics. They also examined the relationship between fasting plasma levels of TMAO and the incident of major adverse cardiovascular events (death, myocardial infarction, or stroke) during a 3-year follow-up in 4007 patients undergoing elective coronary angiography. They found plasma levels of TMAO were markedly suppressed after the administration of antibiotics, and then reappeared after withdrawal of antibiotics. Increased plasma levels of TMAO were associated with an increased risk of a major adverse cardiovascular events.

The relationship between fasting plasma TMAO levels and mortality rate over 5 years in CAD patients was investigated in the *Clinical Outcomes Utilizing Revascularization and Aggressive Drug Evaluation* (COURAGE) trial. The authors looked at fasting plasma TMAO levels and mortality rate in 2,235 CAD patients. They observed a 4-fold increase in the risk of dying in patients with higher plasma TMAO levels, suggesting that elevated plasma TMAO levels present a significant risk in CAD patients.

A study in patients who underwent cardiovascular surgery showed a correlation between serum TMAO levels and the number of blocked coronary arteries. Two independent studies including the Cleveland cohort (n = 530) and Swiss Cohort of ACS patients (n = 1683) found that elevated plasma levels of TMAO, in patients who presented at an emergency room, was an independent risk factor for the development of major adverse cardiac incident. They also concluded that TMAO levels serve as predictors of long-term survival in CAD patients.

A 17-clinical studies meta-analysis with a total of 26,167 patients over a 4–5 years period, reported high TMAO plasma levels were associated with an increased incidence of all-cause mortality. They found an increase of 7.6% in mortality for every 10 μmol/l increase in TMAO levels, suggesting a dose-dependent association between the TMAO levels and cardiovascular mortality. Another study in 3,903 stable CAD patients reported an increase in plasma choline levels (precursor of TMAO) was associated with 1.9-fold increased risk of major adverse cardiac events. However, the increased risk was only associated with an increase in plasma TMAO levels.

10 Polyphenolic Compounds

Polyphenolic compounds fall into several categories according to their structure, including the *stilbenes:* resveratrol, piceatannol, pterostilbene, and the *flavonoids:* apigenin, chrysin, genistein, luteolin, myricetin, and quercetin. The best-known stilbene, resveratrol has been studied for its anti-aging, anti-cancer, anti-oxidant, anti-inflammatory, neuroprotective and cardiovascular properties. The life expectancy of some small organisms has been extended by resveratrol, which is also associated with a slowing down or prevention of cognitive deterioration.

Stilbenes

Resveratrol is classified as a polyphenolic stilbene which is found in peanuts, pistachios, grapes, red and white wine, blueberries, cranberries, cocoa and dark chocolate. Research on resveratrol has focused on such areas as the maintenance of vascular health, prevention of atherosclerosis, and improvement of cardiovascular function. While resveratrol is the best studied, other polyphenols perform similar roles, including apigenin, chrysin, genistein, luteolin, myricetin, and piceatannol. In fact, luteolin and piceatannol are even more potent inhibitors of endothelial cell proliferation.

Unfortunately, resveratrol has a poor bioavailability. The concentration of resveratrol achieved in the blood stream may be significantly lower than the effective doses found in cell and animal studies. Before reaching the target tissue, resveratrol is rapidly degraded in the gastrointestinal tract by gut microbiota. The low bioavailability of resveratrol limits its therapeutic efficiency and may be responsible for the differences in clinical studies. The gap between preclinical and clinical findings may also be attributed to the poor availability requiring higher doses in human compared to rodent studies.

Azorín-Ortuño *et al.*, (2011) studied the pharmacology of resveratrol in the pig, and found only 0.5% of administrated resveratrol was delivered to different organs (e.g., brain, heart, lungs, kidneys, liver, pancreas, spleen, aorta tissue, and urinary bladder) 6 hr. after administration. The peak circulation levels of resveratrol metabolites are achieved 1 hr. post-administration. Most of the resveratrol metabolites are excreted through urine. In rats, resveratrol metabolites were detectable in heart tissues only following a 6-week resveratrol regimen at a dosage of 5 mg per kg of body weight per day. This represents a dose of 455 mg for a 200 lb. individual. The low amount of resveratrol in cardiovascular tissue over time is another problem in determining its therapeutic potential.

Despite the low bioavailability, resveratrol is

readily absorbed by vascular endothelial cells. There is a vast literature describing the molecular mechanisms by which resveratrol affects endothelial cells. Resveratrol acts on monocytes and macrophages as well to modulate the inflammatory response on vascular smooth muscle cells for the regulation of proliferation, and on cardiomyocytes for counteracting high oxidative stress. It has been known since 2002, from the work of Wallerath *et al.* who discovered that resveratrol up-regulates endothelial nitric oxide thereby acting as a vasodilator.

Other studies have also found that resveratrol causes a down regulation of leukocyte adhesion molecules, and increased plasma levels of the anti-inflammatory molecules. However, these studies used variable resveratrol doses, as well as differing treatment periods, and patient populations. Despite these variabilities, these studies suggest resveratrol decreases inflammation in both healthy and patients with cardiovascular disease.

In a study in type-2 diabetics, resveratrol supplementation caused a decrease in arterial stiffness. Moreover, this study also observed a greater effect for those who likely had poor endothelial function before the trial began. This observation was seen in other studies as well suggesting those with worse symptoms before resveratrol supplementation saw a more significant increase than those with fewer clinical symptoms. A study on hypertensive participants given resveratrol, showed that endothelial function improvement was higher for participants that initially had higher low-density lipoproteins (LDL) levels than in participants that had low initial LDL levels

The anti-hypertensive effects of resveratrol have been shown in multiple animal models of hypertension, following treatment of 10 to 320 mg resveratrol/kg body weight/day, for 14 days to 10 weeks, depending on the studies This has been reproduced in clinical studies as well.

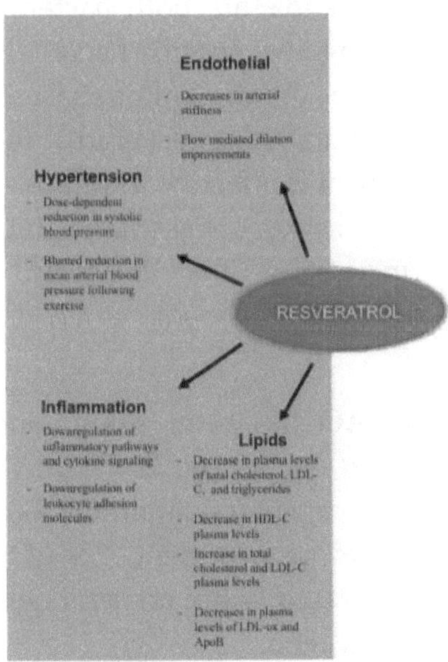

Figure 24: Action of Resveratrol

The mechanisms by which resveratrol decreases blood pressure include the increase in endothelial NO production, reductions in vascular inflammation and oxidative damage in the endothelial cells, and decreased calcium influx. However, the clinical evidence of the effects of resveratrol on blood pressure is not clear cut. Certain clinical studies on resveratrol demonstrated a reduction in systolic blood pressure but not the diastolic pressure. It has been suggested that systolic pressure is more of a risk factor for CVDs than diastolic pressure. However, three meta-analyses publications on the effects of resveratrol on blood pressure have all shown a dose response effect on systolic blood pressure. In these analyses, resveratrol doses higher than 300 mg/d showed a marked reduction on systolic blood pressure reduction.

Resveratrol's major function may be as a prebiotic due its ability to promote the growth of beneficial bacteria and reduce the population of harmful bacteria. Evidence indicates that polyphenols are both bactericidal and bacteriostatic agents against specific bacterial strains, mainly *Clostridia*. In addition, animal-based studies have demonstrated the ability of resveratrol to reduce TMAO levels. Resveratrol is effective in remodeling the microbiota by increasing *Lactobacillus* and *Bifidobacterium* growth, increasing the *Bacteroidetes/Firmicutes* ratio and reducing the *Enterococcus faecalis* growth.

The reduction of TMAO has been shown in randomized clinical studies. In one study, 20 healthy subjects were given resveratrol capsules containing 300 mg twice daily. After 4-weeks of treatment, TMAO levels were significantly decreased with an average decrease of 64% compared to placebo.

Flavonoids

The name *quercetin* is derived from the Latin word *quercetum* meaning "Oak Forest" first isolated in 1857. It is a flavonoid, specifically a subclass called *flavonol*, and is widely distributed in the plant kingdom including apples, berries, brassica vegetables, capers, grapes, onions, spring onions, tea, and tomatoes, as well as in many seeds, nuts, flowers, bark, and leaves. Quercetin is also contained in many medicinal plants, including *Ginkgo biloba, Hypericum perforatum, St John's Wort*, and *elderberry*.

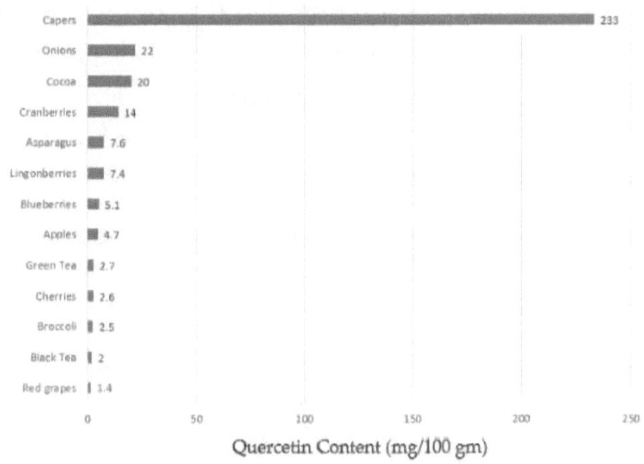

Figure 25: Quercetin content of certain foods (mg/100 gm)

The pharmacokinetics of quercetin in humans suggested very poor oral bioavailability after a single oral dose. Estimated absorption of quercetin glucoside, (the naturally occurring form) ranges from 3% to 17% in healthy individuals receiving a 100 mg dose.

Recent studies indicated that quercetin decreases hyperlipidemia in high-fat fed animals via its effects on the reverse cholesterol transport system. The levels of lipid peroxidation in the plasma and heart, free fatty acid, phospholipid, total cholesterol, and triglyceride in serum were all decreased with quercetin administration.

In addition, Quercetin had significant lowering effects on LDL oxidation. In a study of 93 overweight or obese subjects who were given a daily dose of 150mg quercetin for six weeks showed significant reductions in plasma concentrations of ox-LDL. Several studies done on cell culture revealed that quercetin can reduce ox-LDLs accumulation, foam cell formation, as well as ox-LDLs induced cytotoxicity and calcification. In two clinical studies quercetin significantly reduced plasma concentrations of ox-LDLs.

A meta-analysis of 16 randomized controlled trials published between 2007 and 2017 looked at the effects of quercetin on lipid profiles of patients with metabolic syndrome. The analysis showed quercetin administration resulted in a significant reduction in total and LDL cholesterol, without affecting triglyceride levels. The daily doses and treatment durations used in the trials varied widely (3.12 to 3,000 mg/ day) and from 3 to 12 weeks in duration. Another meta-analysis of 9 humas studies in overweight subjects confirmed that quercetin supplementation significantly reduces LDL cholesterol levels at doses of 250 mg/day or higher. Similar findings were observed in metabolically healthy non-obese adults after an 8-week regimen.

The protective mechanism of quercetin on the cardiovascular system includes reducing systolic blood pressure, diastolic blood pressure, as well as mean arterial pressure. Edwards *et al.* found that, among patients with hypertension, patients who took 730 mg of quercetin per day for 28 days had a decrease in their systolic, diastolic, and mean arterial pressure.

Serban *et al.* (2016) conducted a systematic review of 7 randomized clinical studies published between 1998 and 2014, looking at the effects of quercetin on blood pressure. Their meta-analysis revealed a significant reduction in systemic blood pressure. The doses of quercetin ranged from 100 to 1,000 mg/day. A deeper dive into the data revealed quercetin had no significant benefit in studies lasting less than 8 weeks or doses less than 500 mg/day. Another meta-analysis which included 896 participants across 17 studies showed similar results to those obtained by Serban *et al.* A more recent meta-analysis of 8 studies conducted in patients with metabolic syndrome showed that quercetin significantly reduced systolic blood pressure, yet did not affect diastolic pressure.

The mechanism for the reduction on blood pressure is the decrease in the thickness of the aortic wall via its effect on endothelium nitrogen oxide vasodilation. Quercetin can reverse the endothelial damage caused by excessive nitrogen oxide because of its antioxidant properties, by neutralizing oxygen free radicals, thereby protecting vascular endothelial function. Studies have shown quercetin protects the vascular endothelium from oxidative stress induced by homocysteine by inhibiting lipid peroxidation, protein oxidation, and enzymatic reaction, reducing the level of malondialdehyde.

Studies have demonstrated the ability of quercetin supplementation to reduce areas of atherosclerotic lesions and sizes of plaques. This may be due to alterations in the composition of the gut microbiota and decreased the levels of atherogenic lipid metabolites. Mice that were maintained on a high-fat diet, and treated with quercetin for 12 weeks, exhibited a suppression of body weight gains and a reduction of atherosclerotic lesions. Reduced malondialdehyde levels further indicated the protective effect of quercetin against oxidative stress

Current research suggests there is an antibacterial process by quercetin which mainly includes destroying the cell wall of bacteria and changing the cell permeability, affecting protein synthesis and expression, reducing enzyme activities, and inhibiting nucleic acid synthesis. An analysis of gut microbiota indicate quercetin treatment reduces the abundance of *Verrocomicrobia* and increased microbiome diversity.

About the Author

Thomas Copmann, MS., PhD, has authored over 50 peer-reviewed articles. He holds an MS in Endocrinology and a PhD in Physiology and Post-Doctoral training in Neuroendocrinology. He is currently a consultant to the pharmaceutical industry. He has been active on editorial boards, advisory boards and as a member of boards of directors. He is the former Chair of the Commission on Drugs for Rare Diseases; former Advisor to the National Vaccine Advisory Board. He has served as a scientific advisor to the White House.

References

Abramson J, Wright JM. Are lipid-lowering guidelines evidence-based? Lancet. 2007 Jan 20;369(9557):168-9.

Anderson KM, Castelli WP, Levy D. Cholesterol and mortality. 30 years of follow-up from the Framingham study. JAMA. 1987 Apr 24;257(16):2176-80.

Arnson Y, Itzhaky D, Mosseri M, Barak V, Tzur B, Agmon-Levin N, Amital H. Vitamin D inflammatory cytokines and coronary events: a comprehensive review. Clin Rev Allergy Immunol. 2013 Oct;45(2):236-47.

Azorín-Ortuño M, Yáñez-Gascón MJ, Vallejo F, Pallarés FJ, Larrosa M, Lucas R, Morales JC, Tomás-Barberán FA, García-Conesa MT, Espín JC. Metabolites and tissue distribution of resveratrol in the pig. Mol Nutr Food Res. 2011 Aug;55(8):1154-68.

Barbarawi M, Kheiri B, Zayed Y, Barbarawi O, Dhillon H, Swaid B, Yelangi A, Sundus S, Bachuwa G, Alkotob ML, Manson JE. Vitamin D Supplementation and Cardiovascular Disease Risks in More Than 83 000 Individuals in 21 Randomized Clinical Trials: A Meta-analysis. JAMA Cardiol. 2019 Aug 1;4(8):765-776.

Barter PJ, Caulfield M, Eriksson M, Grundy SM, Kastelein JJ, Komajda M, Lopez-Sendon J, Mosca L, Tardif

JC, Waters DD, Shear CL, Revkin JH, Buhr KA, Fisher MR, Tall AR, Brewer B; ILLUMINATE Investigators. Effects of torcetrapib in patients at high risk for coronary events. N Engl J Med. 2007 Nov 22;357(21):2109-22.

Castelli WP, Anderson K, Wilson PW, Levy D. Lipids and risk of coronary heart disease. The Framingham Study. Ann Epidemiol. 1992 Jan-Mar;2(1-2):23-8.

Dalmeijer GW, van der Schouw YT, Magdeleyns E, Ahmed N, Vermeer C, Beulens JW. The effect of menaquinone-7 supplementation on circulating species of matrix Gla protein. Atherosclerosis. 2012 Dec;225(2):397-402.

Dietary Guidelines for Americans U.S. Department of Agriculture and Health and Human Services, 1980.

Edwards N, Langford-Smith AWW, Wilkinson FL, Alexander MY. Endothelial Progenitor Cells: New Targets for Therapeutics for Inflammatory Conditions With High Cardiovascular Risk. Front Med (Lausanne). 2018 Jul 10;5:200.

Erickson ML, Malin SK, Wang Z, Brown JM, Hazen SL, Kirwan JP. Effects of Lifestyle Intervention on Plasma Trimethylamine N-Oxide in Obese Adults. Nutrients. 2019 Jan 16;11(1):179.

Felton CV, Crook D, Davies MJ, Oliver MF. Dietary polyunsaturated fatty acids and composition of human aortic plaques. Lancet. 1994 Oct 29;344(8931):1195-6.

Finking G, Hanke H. Nikolaj Nikolajewitsch

Anitschkow (1885-1964) established the cholesterol-fed rabbit as a model for atherosclerosis research. Atherosclerosis. 1997;135(1):1-7.

Galvao TF, Brown BH, Hecker PA, O'Connell KA, O'Shea KM, Sabbah HN, Rastogi S, Daneault C, Des Rosiers C, Stanley WC. High intake of saturated fat, but not polyunsaturated fat, improves survival in heart failure despite persistent mitochondrial defects. Cardiovasc Res. 2012 Jan 1;93(1):24-32.

Ghosh S, Molcan E, DeCoffe D, Dai C, Gibson DL. Diets rich in n-6 PUFA induce intestinal microbial dysbiosis in aged mice. Br J Nutr. 2013 Aug 28;110(3):515-23.

Gniwotta C, Morrow JD, Roberts LJ 2nd, Kühn H. Prostaglandin F2-like compounds, F2-isoprostanes, are present in increased amounts in human atherosclerotic lesions. Arterioscler Thromb Vasc Biol. 1997 Nov;17 (11):3236-41.

Harcombe Z, Baker JS, Cooper SM, Davies B, Sculthorpe N, DiNicolantonio JJ, Grace F. Evidence from randomised controlled trials did not support the introduction of dietary fat guidelines in 1977 and 1983: a systematic review and meta-analysis. Open Heart. 2015 Jan 29;2(1):e000196.

Haugsgjerd TR, Egeland GM, Nygård OK, Vinknes KJ, Sulo G, Lysne V, Igland J, Tell GS. Association of dietary vitamin K and risk of coronary heart disease in middle-age adults: the Hordaland Health Study Cohort. BMJ Open. 2020 May 21;10(5):e035953.

KEYS A. Atherosclerosis: a problem in newer public health. J Mt Sinai Hosp N Y. 1953 Jul-Aug;20(2):118-39.

Klose G, März W, Grammer TB, Nitschmann S. Rosuvastatin zur Primärprävention vaskulärer Komplikationen : JUPITER-Studie (Justification for the Use of statins in Prevention: an Intervention Trial Evaluation Rosuvastatin) [Rosuvastatin for primary prevention of vascular events : JUPITER trial (Justification for the Use of statins in Prevention: an Intervention Trial Evaluation Rosuvastatin).]. Internist (Berl). 2010 Jan;51(1):103-106.

Leal-Witt MJ, Llobet M, Samino S, Castellano P, Cuadras D, Jimenez-Chillaron JC, Yanes O, Ramon-Krauel M, Lerin C. Lifestyle Intervention Decreases Urine Trimethylamine N-Oxide Levels in Prepubertal Children with Obesity. Obesity (Silver Spring). 2018 Oct;26(10):1603-1610.

Leren P. The effect of plasma-cholesterol-lowering diet in male survivors of myocardial infarction. A controlled clinical trial. Bull N Y Acad Med. 1968 Aug;44(8):1012-20.

Liao ZL, Zeng BH, Wang W, Li GH, Wu F, Wang L, Zhong QP, Wei H, Fang X. Impact of the Consumption of Tea Polyphenols on Early Atherosclerotic Lesion Formation and Intestinal *Bifidobacteria* in High-Fat-Fed ApoE$^{-/-}$Mice. Front Nutr. 2016 Dec 21;3:42.

Malik M, Suboc TM, Tyagi S, Salzman N, Wang J, Ying R, Tanner MJ, Kakarla M, Baker JE, Widlansky ME. Lactobacillus plantarum 299v Supplementation Improves Vascular Endothelial Function and Reduces Inflammatory Biomarkers in Men With Stable Coronary Artery Disease.

Mancini GB. Overview of the prospective randomized evaluation of the vascular effects of Norvasc (amlodipine) trial: PREVENT. Can J Cardiol. 2000 Jul;16 Suppl D:5D-7D.

Mo R, Zhang X, Yang Y. Effect of probiotics on lipid profiles in hypercholesterolaemic adults: A meta-analysis of randomized controlled trials. Med Clin (Barc). 2019 Jun 21;152(12):473-481.

Mozaffarian D, Rimm EB, Herrington DM. Dietary fats, carbohydrate, and progression of coronary atherosclerosis in postmenopausal women. Am J Clin Nutr. 2004 Nov;80(5):1175-84.

Nakazato R, Gransar H, Berman DS, Cheng VY, Lin FY, Achenbach S, Al-Mallah M, Budoff MJ, Cademartiri F, Callister TQ, Chang HJ, Cury RC, Chinnaiyan K, Chow BJ, Delago A, Hadamitzky M, Hausleiter J, Kaufmann P, Maffei E, Raff G, Shaw LJ, Villines TC, Dunning A, Feuchtner G, Kim YJ, Leipsic J, Min JK. Statins use and coronary artery plaque composition: results from the International Multicenter CONFIRM Registry. Atherosclerosis. 2012 Nov;225(1):148-53.

Naruszewicz M, Johansson ML, Zapolska-Downar D, Bukowska H. Effect of Lactobacillus plantarum 299v on cardiovascular disease risk factors in smokers. Am J Clin Nutr. 2002 Dec;76(6):1249-55.

Newman AB, Naydeck BL, Ives DG, Boudreau RM,

Sutton-Tyrrell K, O'Leary DH, Kuller LH. Coronary artery calcium, carotid artery wall thickness, and cardiovascular disease outcomes in adults 70 to 99 years old. Am J Cardiol. 2008 Jan 15;101(2):186-92.

Niamah AK, Sahi AA, Al-Sharifi ASN. Effect of Feeding Soy Milk Fermented by Probiotic Bacteria on Some Blood Criteria and Weight of Experimental Animals. Probiotics Antimicrob Proteins. 2017 Sep;9(3):284-291.

Nicholls SJ, Borgman M, Nissen SE, Raichlen JS, Ballantyne C, Barter P, Chapman MJ, Erbel R, Libby P. Impact of statins on progression of atherosclerosis: rationale and design of SATURN (Study of Coronary Atheroma by Intravascular Ultrasound: effect of Rosuvastatin versus Atorvastatin). Curr Med Res Opin. 2011 Jun;

27(6):1119-29.

Olijhoek JK, Hajer GR, van der Graaf Y, Dallinga-Thie GM, Visseren FL. The effects of low-dose simvastatin and ezetimibe compared to high-dose simvastatin alone on post-fat load endothelial function in patients with metabolic syndrome: a randomized double-blind crossover trial. J Cardiovasc Pharmacol. 2008 Aug;52(2):145-50.

Page IH, Stare FJ, Corcoran AC, et al. Atherosclerosis and the Fat Content of the Diet: Report to the AHA and to the American Society for the Study of Arteriosclerosis the Nutrition Committee of the Council on Community Service and Education of the AHA and others. Circulation. 1957;16(2):163-178.

Pedersen TR, Kjekshus J, Berg K, Haghfelt T, Faergeman O, Faergeman G, Pyörälä K, Miettinen T, Wilhelmsen L, Olsson AG, Wedel H; Scandinavian Simvastatin Survival Study Group. Randomised trial of cholesterol lowering in 4444 patients with coronary heart disease: the Scandinavian Simvastatin Survival Study (4S). 1994. Atheroscler Suppl. 2004 Oct;5(3):81-7.

Petursson H, Sigurdsson JA, Bengtsson C, Nilsen TI, Getz L. Is the use of cholesterol in mortality risk algorithms in clinical guidelines valid? Ten years prospective data from the Norwegian HUNT 2 study. J Eval Clin Pract. 2012 Feb;18(1):159-68.

Radovanovic S, Savic-Radojevic A, Pljesa-Ercegovac M, Djukic T, Suvakov S, Krotin M, Simic DV, Matic M, Radojicic Z, Pekmezovic T, Simic T. Markers of oxidative damage and antioxidant enzyme activities as predictors of morbidity and mortality in patients with chronic heart failure. J Card Fail. 2012 Jun;18(6):493-501.

Randrianarisoa E, Lehn-Stefan A, Wang X, Hoene M, Peter A, Heinzmann SS, Zhao X, Königsrainer I, Königsrainer A, Balletshofer B, Machann J, Schick F, Fritsche A, Häring HU, Xu G, Lehmann R, Stefan N. Relationship of Serum Trimethylamine N-Oxide (TMAO) Levels with early Atherosclerosis in Humans. Sci Rep. 2016 May 27;6:26745.

Ramsden CE, Zamora D, Leelarthaepin B, Majchrzak-Hong SF, Faurot KR, Suchindran CM, Ringel A, Davis JM, Hibbeln JR. Use of dietary linoleic acid for secondary prevention of coronary heart disease and death: evaluation of recovered data from the Sydney Diet Heart Study and updated meta-analysis. BMJ. 2013 Feb 4;346:e8707.

Ranque B, Menet A, Boutouyrie P, Diop IB, Kingue S, Diarra M, N'Guetta R, Diallo D, Diop S, Diagne I, Sanogo I, Tolo A, Chelo D, Wamba G, Gonzalez JP, Abough'elie C, Diakite CO, Traore Y, Legueun G, Deme-Ly I, Faye BF, Seck M, Kouakou B, Kamara I, Le Jeune S, Jouven X. Arterial Stiffness Impairment in Sickle Cell Disease Associated With Chronic Vascular Complications: The Multinational African CADRE Study. Circulation. 2016 Sep 27;134(13):923-33.

Raygan F, Ostadmohammadi V, Bahmani F, Asemi Z. The effects of vitamin D and probiotic co-supplementation on mental health parameters and metabolic status in type 2 diabetic patients with coronary heart disease: A randomized, double-blind, placebo-controlled trial. Prog Neuropsychopharmacol Biol Psychiatry. 2018 Jun 8;84(Pt A):50-55.

Rose, GA., Thomson, WB., and Williams, RT. Corn Oil in Treatment of Ischaemic Heart Disease.. Br Med J. 1965 Jun 12;1(5449):1531-3.

Saremi A, Bahn G, Reaven PD; VADT Investigators. Progression of vascular calcification is increased with statin use in the Veterans Affairs Diabetes Trial (VADT). Diabetes Care. 2012 Nov;35(11):2390-2.

Satilmis S, Celik O, Biyik I, Ozturk D, Celik K, Akın F, Ayca B, Yalcin B, Dagdelen S. Association between serum vitamin D levels and subclinical coronary athero-sclerosis and plaque burden/composition in young adult population. Bosn J Basic Med Sci. 2015 Feb 8;15(1):67-72.

Seibert E, Lehmann U, Riedel A, Ulrich C, Hirche F, Brandsch C, Dierkes J, Girndt M, Stangl GI. Vitamin D_3 supplementation does not modify cardiovascular risk profile of adults with inadequate vitamin D status. Eur J Nutr. 2017 Mar;56(2):621-634.

Serban MC, Sahebkar A, Zanchetti A, Mikhailidis DP, Howard G, Antal D, Andrica F, Ahmed A, Aronow WS, Muntner P, Lip GY, Graham I, Wong N, Rysz J, Banach M; Lipid and Blood Pressure Meta-analysis Collaboration (LBPMC) Group. Effects of Quercetin on Blood Pressure: A Systematic Review and Meta-Analysis of Randomized Controlled Trials. J Am Heart Assoc. 2016 Jul 12;5(7):e002713.

Shaw LJ, Berman DS, Maron DJ, Mancini GB, Hayes SW, Hartigan PM, Weintraub WS, O'Rourke RA, Dada M, Spertus JA, Chaitman BR, Friedman J, Slomka P, Heller GV, Germano G, Gosselin G, Berger P, Kostuk WJ, Schwartz RG, Knudtson M, Veledar E, Bates ER, McCallister B, Teo KK, Boden WE; COURAGE Investigators. Optimal medical therapy with or without percutaneous coronary intervention to reduce ischemic burden: results from the Clinical Outcomes Utilizing Revascularization and Aggressive Drug Evaluation (COURAGE) trial nuclear substudy. Circulation. 2008 Mar 11;117(10):1283-91.

Sokol SI, Tsang P, Aggarwal V, Melamed ML, Srinivas VS. Vitamin D status and risk of cardiovascular events: lessons learned via systematic review and meta-analysis. Cardiol Rev. 2011 Jul-Aug;19(4):192-201.

Sutherland WH, de Jong SA, Hessian PA, Williams MJ. Ingestion of native and thermally oxidized polyunsaturated fats acutely increases circulating numbers of endothelial microparticles. Metabolism. 2010 Mar; 59(3): 446-53.

Tang WH, Wang Z, Levison BS, Koeth RA, Britt EB, Fu X, Wu Y, Hazen SL. Intestinal microbial metabolism of phosphatidylcholine and cardiovascular risk. N Engl J Med. 2013 Apr 25;368(17):1575-84.

The Lipid Research Clinics Coronary Primary Prevention Trial results. I. Reduction in incidence of coronary heart disease. JAMA. 1984 Jan 20;251(3):351-64.

Trombold JC, Moellering RC Jr, Kagan A. Epidemiological aspects of coronary heart disease and cerebrovascular disease: the Honolulu Heart Program. Hawaii Med J. 1966 Jan-Feb;25(3):231-4.

United States, U. States, Congress, C., Senate, S., & Select Committee on Nutrition and Human Needs, S. Committee on Nutrition and Human Needs. Dietary goals for the United States.

Waddington EI, Croft KD, Sienuarine K, Latham B, Puddey IB. Fatty acid oxidation products in human atherosclerotic plaque: an analysis of clinical and histopathological correlates. Atherosclerosis. 2003 Mar;167(1):111-20.

Wallerath T, Deckert G, Ternes T, Anderson H, Li H, Witte K, Förstermann U. Resveratrol, a polyphenolic phytoalexin present in red wine, enhances expression and activity of endothelial nitric oxide synthase. Circulation. 2002 Sep 24;106(13):1652-8.

Yam D, Eliraz A, Berry EM. Diet and disease--the Israeli paradox: possible dangers of a high omega-6 polyunsaturated fatty acid diet. Isr J Med Sci. 1996 Nov;32(11):1134-43.

Yu D, Shu XO, Rivera ES, Zhang X, Cai Q, Calcutt MW, Xiang YB, Li H, Gao YT, Wang TJ, Zheng W. Urinary Levels of Trimethylamine-N-Oxide and Incident Coronary Heart Disease: A Prospective Investigation Among Urban Chinese Adults. J Am Heart Assoc. 2019 Jan 8;8(1):e010606.

Zeisel SH, Wishnok JS, Blusztajn JK. Formation of methylamines from ingested choline and lecithin. J Pharmacol Exp Ther. 1983 May;225(2):320-4.

www.ingramcontent.com/pod-product-compliance
Lightning Source LLC
Chambersburg PA
CBHW031403250726
48656CB00002B/537